MW01062041

The Cochrane Collaboration
MEDICINE'S BEST-KEPT SECRET

The Cochrane Collaboration

MEDICINE'S BEST-KEPT SECRET

ALAN CASSELS

Foreword by
SIR IAIN CHALMERS

Illustrations by
JEREMY GORDANEER

PUBLISHING HOUSE

To Jini:
The first ever awardee
of the Chris Silagy Prize

PUBLISHING HOUSE

151 Howe Street, Victoria BC Canada V8V 4K5

The Cochrane Collaboration:
Medicine's Best-Kept Secret
    978-1-927755-30-3 (trade paperback)
    978-1-927755-31-0 (kindle/mobi ebook)
    978-1-927755-32-7 (epub ebook)

Cataloguing information available from
Library and Archives Canada.
Printed on acid-free paper.
Agio Publishing House is a socially responsible
enterprise, measuring success on a triple-bottom-
line basis.
10 9 8 7 6 5 4 3 2 1

TABLE OF CONTENTS

Sir Iain Chalmers

IN 1972, when Archie Cochrane published his seminal work, *Effectiveness and Efficiency: Random Reflections on Health Services*,[1] he asked a vital question: how can we have rational health services if we don't know which of the things being done are useful and which are useless or possibly even harmful?

Archie went on to indicate where one might start to find the answers. He said that not all professional opinions are equal: some are informed by mediocre or no research; others are supported by more rigorous research, such as unbiased treatment comparisons made within randomized trials.

Being introduced to randomized trials in Archie's book was, for me, like being given a compass to negotiate the jungle of incompatible clinical opinions that I faced as a junior doctor. I started looking out for reports of randomized trials in my chosen field, obstetrics. The bibliographic databases at that time hadn't indexed these studies satisfactorily, which meant searching journals for them 'by hand'. A scheme was outlined for evaluating the studies found. Over the next ten years we extended our searches to the point at which we felt able to begin analyzing similar studies together, sometimes combining their results to reduce the likelihood of being misled by the play of chance.

In this book by bestselling author and health policy researcher

Alan Cassels, you'll learn that Archie Cochrane judged my specialty – obstetrics – the most unscientific in medicine! That jibe helped to provide the impetus to tackle this situation, and about a hundred of us from around the world collaborated to show what could be done. Archie Cochrane himself recognized our progress the year before he died. He referred to our collection of systematic reviews of controlled trials of care during pregnancy and childbirth "a real milestone in the history of randomized trials and in the evaluation of care," and expressed his hope that it would be "widely copied by other specialties."

This presented a new challenge. Why shouldn't the approach we had used successfully for maternity care be extended across all of health care? The key to establishing the international collaboration needed to take up Archie's new challenge was to involve people who were generous-spirited, who respected other people's views, and who were team builders.

In this book you will read about some of these people, and others who have contributed to the collaboration over the past 20 years. Cochrane's name was built into the initiative when a Cochrane Centre was established in Oxford in 1992, and the Centre convened a meeting the following year at which the international Cochrane Collaboration was founded. The Collaboration now has well over 30,000 contributors in over a hundred countries, who prepare, maintain and disseminate thousands of systematic reviews of research evidence relevant to improving health care. One result of reviewing such a mass of research is that it has laid bare the poor quality and irrelevance to patients and clinicians of much medical research.

I left the Cochrane Collaboration ten years after helping to establish it, and I have deliberately not tried to keep myself informed about its development. However, I was asked to give the 1st Archie Cochrane Lecture at the Cochrane Colloquium in Quebec City in 2013, so I had to do some informal research to help me prepare my talk. I began the talk by reminding my audience of the principal motivation for many if not most of those who contribute to the Collaboration: when decisions in health care are not informed by up-to-date, systematic reviews of research, patients suffer and sometimes die.

Keeping reviews up to date is a particular challenge for the Collaboration because – uniquely – its publicly stated mission is to prepare *and maintain* systematic reviews of treatments. This is also the Collaboration's 'Achilles heel'. Cochrane reviews have earned a deserved reputation for being of generally high quality, but some of them don't live up to the resulting expectations, and they often take an age to move through the preparation, publication and updating processes. I acknowledged that the Collaboration was very aware of these criticisms and was taking them seriously.

I made clear in my talk that I appreciated that the Cochrane Collaboration had been one of the principal contributors to the global explosion in systematic reviews over the previous 20 years; had promulgated the ethical and scientific principles of systematic reviews; trained tens of thousands of people in systematic review methods; established novel editorial systems for assuring quality in preparing reviews; created and made publicly available the best bibliographic source of reports of controlled trials in the world, as well as the most widely used software for preparing systematic reviews; and had established a network of methods groups and a database of methodological research.

This was all well and good, but given the burgeoning production of systematic reviews by people outside the Cochrane Collaboration, and the development of sources of information other than Cochrane reviews, was there anything special about the Collaboration? Indeed, were others providing the same or a better service to patients and health professionals more efficiently?

I have no sentimentality about the Cochrane Collaboration. But if the organization didn't exist, something like it would need to be invented to serve the information needs of patients and health professionals. If that could be achieved through means other than the Cochrane Collaboration, I wouldn't shed any tears at the demise of the organization. However, the Collaboration does remain unique in some important respects. It registers the titles of its planned reviews and publishes the protocols of reviews being prepared. It has developed the editorial and technical infrastructure to assure quality and to update and correct its reviews. And it has established exceptional international coverage.

I suggested in my talk that one of the Collaboration's most precious features has been its tradition of self-criticism. One of the things I remember with pleasure about the founding Colloquium in Oxford in 1993 was that there weren't any bull-shitters there: bullshitters are uncomfortable in the Cochrane Collaboration because, however distinguished they may be, they get challenged, sometimes by very 'junior' people, if they manifest the arrogance that is not uncommon among senior doctors. There is a strong tradition of challenging authority within the Cochrane Collaboration, and there's even an annual prize for the best (evidence-based) criticism of the Collaboration – whether self-criticism or criticism from outside.

After interviewing me for nearly two hours on the origins of the Cochrane Collaboration, Alan Cassels ended by asking me what I am most proud of. I said that, "Pride is not something which I find comes particularly easily; but if you had asked me instead what I am most pleased about, I would say that it is the self-criticism and generosity of spirit among the people contributing to the Cochrane Collaboration. These are the organization's most important qualities."

In the pages of this book you will learn about some of the generous-spirited people who continue to do their best, despite the frustrations, to ensure that the Cochrane Collaboration "serves the people" with timely, trustworthy research information relevant to choices in health care.

Preface

IF YOU read this preface as part of a book printed on paper, then consider it a minor miracle. This book almost never got published.

For more than a decade, I had been an outside observer of the Cochrane Collaboration, an occasional lurker at its annual Colloquium. This often required a trek to some exotic locale such as Keystone, Colorado or Melbourne, Australia to meet the people responsible for the best there is in healthcare research. My lurking at those meetings must have been noticed. The Cochrane leadership approached me in 2011 and asked me to consider writing a book about the organization.

The first sentiment that came to my mind was the glib expression of Groucho Marx: *Did I really want to belong to any club that would have me as a member?* I had meetings and teleconferences with the organizers, and they explained that a book could showcase the "social history" of the organization and help to mark its 20th-anniversary celebrations taking place in Quebec City, Canada, in September, 2013.

I felt a little reluctant – I'm not the showcasing type. I'm a hopeless failure at PR and typically don't do promotional writing, because often there is little worth showcasing. It didn't help that "social history" sounded a little pompous, and I was pretty sure I didn't have a clue what it was or why anyone would actually care. In hindsight, the term "social history" was a misnomer: to academics it means something very specific, and this was not the book I wrote.

I felt pretty confident that maybe the world didn't need a book about the Cochrane Collaboration. There were already so many stories – legends really – about many of the characters who struggled to create a movement known as evidence-based health care. Many of those characters – including quirky activists and punctilious academics, some who were the early founders of the Cochrane Collaboration – inhabited stories that almost reach the status of folk tales in the world of medical research.

Then there was the irony of creating something in print – a book, on paper, with a cover – which was not lost on me. The Cochrane Collaboration has always been a virtual organization. Its enormous, influential output has always been electronic. Cochrane (which is what the Collaboration is now called after the latest round of rebranding) began at roughly the same time as computers were becoming common in homes and offices, and we began communicating through them.

Paper has always been superfluous while the thousands of systematic reviews of healthcare interventions produced by the Cochrane Collaboration – what some would call the very bedrock of what we can say we really *know* in health care – are in computers, accessible anywhere to anyone with internet access. Those reviews, plus thousands more pages describing the methods and the careful documentation that support the work of the Collaboration, existed in cyberspace long before anyone ever used the term "in the cloud."

After much thought, I agreed to write the book because the leadership gave me some measure of solace that I, as a writer, wouldn't starve in the process. I did actually find the beginnings of the Collaboration to be a very compelling, critically important story worth telling. But most of all, I did want to showcase this organization, which, apart from healthcare professionals and researchers, almost no one on the planet has ever really heard of.

I'm naturally attracted to those who fight against corruption and misleading medical research and the books I have written tend to highlight these struggles. The Collaboration is a big and diverse – some might even say overly bureaucratic these days – organization but within it there are people who have done and continue to do remarkable things, and display incredible courage and conviction in fighting off the adverse influences of money and power on health research. They have often won huge victories that influence everyone on the planet who seeks health care. Not bad for an organization that is largely unheard of.

Quite simply, I figured that this 'secret' organization was making the world a better place, and it would help if more people knew about it. Hey, maybe this was a club I *did* want to belong to! If these accomplishments needed a megaphone, then maybe I was the one who could give it to them.

EVERY DAY around the globe, people grapple with illness, not knowing if a recommended drug, test, or medical procedure will ultimately improve their lives, make no difference, or hasten their demise. Among the sheer variety of medical questions we will ask at one time in our lives, there will always be, for all of us, the hardest question of all: "Is there anywhere I can go for reliable, trustworthy information about how to treat my condition?"

If you have never given a second thought to medical research and have never tried to second-guess your doctor's orders, then this book might rattle your worldview. It is not only about one of medicine's best-kept secrets, but also about the organization that exposes secrets – especially those related to what we know and what we don't know about health care.

Today, more than 20 years after its creation, many doctors, nurses, researchers, and public health officials who make big decisions affecting the health care we receive consult the Cochrane Collaboration. It is a network of more than 30,000 people around the world, mostly volunteers, who collect and summarize research on healthcare interventions. For most of the world, Cochrane works in the shadows, its members working largely in obscurity, trying to accumulate knowledge to help people decide if the health care offered will truly help – and not harm – them.

You may rightly ask, "Don't medical people always offer what's going to help and not harm their patients?"

No. They don't.

In fact, what they currently don't know is alarming.

Think of healthcare interventions as a pie sliced into thirds. The first third contains all those healthcare interventions – pharmaceuticals, surgeries and tests, for example —underpinned by reliable evidence. They have been fairly studied and we can say, with more or less certainty, that they "work." Call that piece of pie *evidence-based.*

The next third of pie comprises all those interventions that are either insufficiently studied or where proof is unknown; that we think are likely to help but for which there is not yet definitive proof that the benefits exceed the harms.

The final third contains all interventions for which the available evidence shows that the drug or procedure is likely harmful. And. We. Should. Stop. Doing. It.

Feelings of confusion may turn to suspicion as you wonder, *"But how do I know which piece of pie is being served up by my doctor?"* If you find this thought uncomfortable, that's a good sign. You might have just had an "aha" moment similar to the one that struck Scottish physician Archie Cochrane.

He wondered, in a very public way, why his profession wasn't systematically looking for reliable proof behind what he and his fellow doctors were offering their patients. He saw this as an unconscionable state of affairs, so he threw down a gauntlet at doctors, shaming them into action.

That gauntlet was picked up by Dr. (now Sir) Iain Chalmers, a young British obstetrician whose incredible zeal for the truth concerning medical approaches to pregnancy and childbirth fuelled the beginnings of this organization. He named it after his mentor and challenger.

That "aha" moment – as I show in the first chapter – had the power to change a person's life. It changed my life, too, though not in a way I'd expected.

Over the two years I spent researching and writing this book, I traveled to Madrid, Oxford, Paris and Quebec City. I carried out more than 160 interviews with people both inside and outside the Cochrane Collaboration. Those interviews were video recorded and made part of the 20-year Cochrane anniversary celebrations, and many are now viewable on the Cochrane website www.cochrane.org. I talked to those critical of the Collaboration, those who lead it, and many who are part of the 30,000-or-so volunteers who work to make health care more evidence-based, more rational, and more lifesaving.

In January of 2013, shortly after I handed in a 100,000-word manuscript to Wiley, the Cochrane Library's London-based publisher who was lined up to publish this book, Wiley's executives got cold feet and withdrew from the project. Apparently they too were thinking like Groucho, not wanting to be part of a club that would have Alan Cassels as a member. I understood this in hindsight: big companies that worry about their "brand" don't want anyone tinkering with it.

There are more layers of politics to this organization than one can ever contemplate. Many of the bigwigs in the Collaboration are skilled researchers and clinicians, but also skilled politicians, steeped in the myriad power struggles that make up modern health care. In an organization where every snort or wheeze about medical evidence holds huge consequences for the gargantuan business of health care out in the real world, one couldn't have some renegade tampering with "the brand."

From its early days as a rebel band of misfits that would criticize their superiors with the demand, "Show us the evidence!" the Collaboration has grown into a worldwide beacon of research excellence. "What does Cochrane say?" is often the first question any researcher would ask before setting out to find the answers to how well any healthcare intervention is supported by evidence. The early zeal that begat this organization has morphed. The cliché now routinely bandied about among the Collaboration's old timers: "We used to fight the establishment, but now, we *ARE* the establishment."

What you hold in your hands is a somewhat pared-down version of my original manuscript, which is a slice of how things looked in the years 2012 and 2013, as the Collaboration was planning for and celebrating its 20th anniversary. When people inside the organization read this, they will say it's dated. Things have changed. People have moved to different positions. The world has continued revolving on its axis. I get that, but please accept this as how things looked to me, the lurker, as this organization was turning 20. I hope that you, my dear reader, will marvel at the stories of the people in this book who I believe have created something truly remarkable. In these pages you will meet some of the finest healthcare champions alive today, many of them still toiling in obscurity, against the greatest of odds for the benefit of humankind, under the banner of Cochrane.

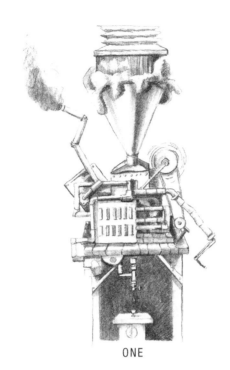

ONE

An "aha" Moment

He has developed concepts, grins
Obscenely at your Royal bulletins,
Possesses what he calls a will
Which challenges your power to kill.

— E.J. Pratt, *The Truant*[2]

NANCY OWENS remembers when she first heard the secret. It happened about 15 years ago, when looking for a job. She was living in Oxford, England, when she saw an advertisement for an administrative position with the Cochrane research group examining the evidence around treatments for people with schizophrenia.

Originally from Boston, Owens hasn't lost her Boston accent, despite having spent much of her adult life in the UK, Australia and the American Midwest[3]. Now based in Canberra, she is quick to admit that she is "not a medical person or a scientist." She wasn't sure what to expect when she saw the job description. "My experience with health care was completely as a consumer, and when I started to understand what the Collaboration was all about – looking for and summarizing evidence for health care – my initial reaction was, 'You mean medicine's *not* evidence-based? That's not how doctors make decisions about treatment?'"

Owens had always assumed that what lay behind doctors' decisions was high-quality research. What did it mean, then, in the words of the Collaboration maxim, "to provide the best evidence for health care"? She was about to find out.

This "aha" moment might cause you to shut down, saying, "I don't want to think about this." Or it might draw you in; make you want to know more and understand more clearly what really underpins healthcare decisions. Owens' "aha" moment drew her in, and that first Cochrane job has grown into a career.

In the course of her work, Nancy Owens not only discovered medicine's best-kept secret, but also became intrinsic to an organization trying to draw itself out of the shadows of research obscurity into the full light of social media. The Cochrane Collaboration has been and remains a secret to the lay public who give little thought to the intricacies of healthcare research and to the many arguments concerning what is and what is not valid medical science.

The greater secret is that there is much falsity and foolishness in medicine today. There are many ways people – including healthcare practitioners themselves – are misled, and many people who claim to have "the answer" cannot support their opinions with evidence. Few of us like to face the fact that much of health care today is not based on solid research and good science.

To uncover the BS requires skilled, disciplined people dedicated to truth-seeking; constantly willing to deconstruct their own assumptions and biases. That is at the heart of the Cochrane Collaboration.

Today, Nancy Owens is Cochrane's web content and social media editor, helping to lead the Collaboration into the world of social media. One of her many tasks is to analyze the organization's interactions with its various audiences, ensuring that "we always benefit from having more people, more diversity, more perspectives." In her words, "It's also about engaging people, whether it's engaging them to the point where they are looking at what's in the *Cochrane Library* that might apply to them, or enticing them to get more involved with the Collaboration in one of the many ways they can get involved."

Owens is a promoter of the Cochrane Collaboration, and she's a user of the *Cochrane Library*, which includes more than 5,000 systematic reviews on a wide range of healthcare topics. Eight years ago, when her mother was diagnosed with colon cancer – a potentially life-threatening condition – Owens, like any daughter would, was reaching for whatever lifebuoys she could find. She went first to the *Cochrane Library*[4] (www.thecochranelibrary.com) and gathered information from reviews in the database.

An individual study of a drug or other therapy found on the internet is an island of limited use. The *Cochrane Library* stores systematic reviews – systematic collections and assessments of all the relevant research to answer a question: this is research *in context*. In the words of Iain Chalmers, a co-founder of The Cochrane Collaboration, "People don't need islands unconnected to any continent. They want something which tells them: What does it mean?"

Owens felt reassured to find that her mother's treatment protocol was in line with the latest available evidence, but she went further than that, even asking her mother's doctors if she could see the citation that supported the treatment they were using. As she said, "That's something that, in the past, I never would have been able to do."

What she felt most was a sense of confidence, knowing that she could help her mother by being a scout for reliable information. Thanks to the *Cochrane Library*, she could become familiar with her mother's treatment protocol, what it was supposed to achieve, based on the best evidence at the time, and what was supposed to happen next.

She recalls, "It also meant that I felt comfortable about trying to communicate that information to my mother in a way that I knew she would be able to absorb." She describes what all of us have probably experienced: "When you're talking to doctors, quite frequently, you don't really take anything in." Owens, however, was able to take accurate information to her mother and "go over it again and again with her later."

Owens knew where to look for high-quality information because she was already part of the Cochrane Collaboration. But who put this information together? What motivates them, and what challenges do they face? Above all – this is the fundamental Cochrane question – is there good evidence that the healthcare advice we're getting is likely to help and not harm?

Try taking that question for a test drive. See how it makes you think about your doctor's next recommendation for a treatment, a screening test, or a vaccine.

False Hope

On October 14, 1993, the day before the Cochrane Collaboration held its inaugural meeting in Oxford, a meeting of a different sort was held across the Atlantic Ocean, in Washington, DC. A busload of 70 women had driven the 260-or-so miles from Durham, North Carolina, to Capitol Hill to meet with members of Congress. They went to argue that President Clinton's healthcare reforms should include paying for expensive treatments for people enrolled in clinical trials. These weren't just any women. Every single one of them had received a controversial breast cancer treatment called high-dose chemotherapy with autologous bone marrow transplantation (HDC/ABMT), which could cost between $100,000 and $200,000 per patient.

These women were foot soldiers in the war on cancer, survivors of the second most deadly cancer for women, and they believed that HDC/ABMT had saved their lives. So they made the pilgrimage to Washington to meet the lawmakers and to act as living testimony to ensure that no woman with breast cancer would be denied access to this treatment.

There was, however, one problem: There was no credible scientific evidence that HDC/ABMT was better than, or even as effective as, conventional treatment. There were suggestions that it could even be worse, making more women suffer and die than those treated conventionally.

The breast cancer community was deeply divided on this treatment. Some women, swayed by the testimonials of survivors, demanded that the treatment be available to all. There were many vested interests behind this lobbying effort: the lawyers who represented breast cancer sufferers, the drug companies who sold the treatment, the physicians who staked their reputations on it, and the patient advocates who were convinced that the treatment gave them a second chance; that it had saved their lives.

Other advocates said that the procedure shouldn't be offered outside of randomized controlled trials (RCTs) and that, without reliable science behind the procedure, no one could be sure if women were being helped instead of harmed.

An RCT is considered the gold standard of reliable evidence. Did the HDC/ABMT extend and improve the lives of women with breast cancer or not? The best way to determine this uses a control group, which can help reduce bias and the likelihood that there might be other factors influencing the outcome. An RCT reduces bias by assigning patients at random either to a treatment group or to a comparison group, with neither patients nor study officials knowing who will get what before the allocation is made.

One of those pushing for RCTs was Kay Dickersin, an epidemiologist from Baltimore, and a breast cancer survivor herself, who made an impassioned plea for "science-based, evidence-based medicine."[5]

Dickersin was a founding member of the National Breast Cancer Coalition (NBCC), formed in 1991, which considers itself a strongly evidence-based organization. Dickersin wasn't considering the treatment for herself. As someone who had studied clinical trials, she was there at the table when the NBCC was grappling with the issue of HDC/ABMT, as well as mammography, and trying to decide what position the organization should take.

It was not at all clear whether HDT/ABMT represented an overall benefit for women, despite how strongly and how vocally women said they wanted access to it. Dickersin emphasized that there are many ways to bias science, and that it was outrageous to promote such a treatment without sound evidence that it was improving the lives of women exposed to it.

She was right to be skeptical. And her demands that the procedure be studied in a rigorous trial were eventually satisfied. By the time HDC/ABMT was definitively studied and evaluated, six years had passed. Somewhere between 23,000 and 40,000 women had received this treatment, costing US taxpayers and private citizens several billion dollars. The evidence was definitive, and damning. It showed that women given HDC/ABMT fared considerably *worse* than those on conventional therapy. It was found to seriously impair those patients' quality of life, as well as increasing their risk of death.

The book that documents this debacle, *False Hope: Bone*

Marrow Transplantation for Breast Cancer[6], details the story of how both physicians' and patients' enthusiasm for new treatments, bolstered by captivating media stories of survival, consumer advocacy, legal challenges, and even fraudulent science, all conspired against amassing the evidence. And women paid, suffered, and died because of it.

Too Many Cautionary Tales Unheeded

Kay Dickersin called the HDC/ABMT fiasco "a cautionary tale of what happens when our hopes for a medical breakthrough lead us to press for access to it too soon." She has seen many similar tales unfold over the years. Dickersin is currently Director of the Center for Clinical Trials at the Johns Hopkins Bloomberg School of Public Health and Director of the US Cochrane Center. As one of the American founders of the Cochrane Collaboration, she is undoubtedly one of the most avid promoters of evidence-based health care (EBHC) in the USA.

At its heart, EBHC is simple. In Dickersin's words, EBHC is "healthcare practice that is based on integrating knowledge gained from the best available research evidence, clinical expertise, and patients' values and circumstances." To her, EBHC is not just some kind of medical nonsense jargon; it is "one of the most important milestones in the history of medicine."

In 2007, in a special issue of the *British Medical Journal (BMJ)* looking at medical milestones since 1840 (when the *BMJ* began publishing), she and two colleagues consider what seems an obvious question: "It is curious, even shocking, that the adjective 'evidence-based' is needed. The public must wonder on what basis medical decisions are made otherwise. Is it intuition? Magic?"[7] They go on to note that without an "evidence base" for medicine, none of the *BMJ*'s 14 other noteworthy milestones, including antibiotics, vaccinations, and anesthesia, would have been achieved.

Dickersin and her colleagues then invite readers into a thought experiment: What would a world without EBHC look like? They provide some examples:

+ many more women with early breast cancer getting total breast removal instead of choosing the less-invasive lumpectomy and radiation
+ many more premature babies dying because women didn't get a simple corticosteroid treatment while in labor
+ more women getting HDC/ABMT and dying earlier.

When facing an illness, I think, most of us hope that things will get better; that the health care we receive will help us to recover and live well until we are old. But merely hoping that a treatment will work is not a viable strategy. We also have to ask for proof that healthcare treatment offered is likely to confer benefit and not harm.

People like Dickersin, who have contributed to the Cochrane Collaboration's many achievements, have seen the devastation that results from false hope. Rather than make them despair, some find that it motivates them to do more: to seek out, to analyze, and sometimes to demand high-quality research. Dickersin is among those constantly challenging physicians and patients to become active questioners, always asking, "Is there good evidence for this practice?"

Ubiquitously Pink

If you've spent any time in the USA, Canada or the United Kingdom during October, then you've probably noticed the ubiquitous pinkness. People wear pink ribbons on their clothes and their cars; pink ribbons are on many products in stores; you can buy pink buckets of Kentucky Fried Chicken, and even see American football players wearing pink gloves. On the first day of October, one of the most famous buildings in the USA, the White House, becomes the Pink House, signaling the beginning of the annual Breast Cancer Awareness Month. A consortium of cancer agencies and breast cancer advocates have branded the entire month pink as a way to raise awareness and money.

While it is easy to be cynical about such corporate-backed campaigns (one critic sniped that "breast cancer has become a product, not just a disease"[8]), one of the most important messages that comes with all the pinkification is that women must be vigilant about their breast health and submit to routine mammography screening.

Mammography screening uses X-rays to find tumors in the breasts. It is recommended annually or semi-annually for women after the age of 40 or 50. (The optimal age to start depends on whom you ask.) There have been breast cancer screening programs in place in nations around the world for decades, but what there hasn't been is good evidence that mammography screening programs actually save lives.

We *believe* that they save lives. We are told by influential organizations including the American Cancer Society (ACS) that screening is the right thing to do. The ACS used to run advertisements in magazines targeting women 35 and older with the slogan, "If you haven't had a mammogram, you need more than your breasts examined,"[9] implying that avoiding mammography screening meant you were crazy.

Medical screening for many varieties of disease is popular in the USA, yet no screening program is bigger, more widely promoted, and perhaps more controversial than the screening program that focuses on women's breasts. The notoriety of mammography is understandable in light of the toll taken by the disease. After lung cancer, it is the most common type of cancer death for women in the USA.

Like those advocating for HDC/ABMT, thousands of enthusiastic survivors in the USA advocate breast cancer awareness, many saying that they owe their lives to mammography.

According to BreastCancer.org, "as of Jan. 1, 2009, there were about 2,747,459 women alive in the United States with a history of breast cancer," a figure that includes women being treated and women who have had cancer and are now disease-free.[10]

Many women who have gone through breast cancer have come out the other side transformed into foot soldiers in the War on Cancer, spreading the message that women must be vigilant and get early and frequent mammography screening if they want to save their own lives.

Kay Dickersin is one of those nearly three million American breast cancer survivors, but she's unlikely to wear pink and make appeals to her friends to get mammograms to save their lives. She has seen far too many women enthusiastically endorse procedures and treatments that, when better studied, were proven harmful. Apart from the muscle of a lobby that can turn the White House into the Pink House, there is the Cochrane Collaboration, continually (some might say tirelessly) asking for the evidence.

Mammography is a procedure that millions of otherwise healthy women submit to every year. Kay Dickersin said, "Cochrane has kept on the radar screen the fact that mammography, even if it works, isn't a great method for detecting early breast cancer or for preventing death, that there's overdiagnosis, and that people are treated who don't need to be treated." And in addition, it's "a huge source of income and expenditure" – money that, in the absence of proof that screening programs save lives, might be better employed.

As someone who has been through breast cancer treatment, Dickersin is aware of its serious and life-altering consequences. But she also thinks of the big picture. Mammography is only one type of medical screening of many being promoted to the general public. That makes her ask, "There are more and more screening tests, so what are we going to do? Are we going to keep adding them on? Or are we going to think about what sort of impact they have on health? It's not just a matter of are they accurate or not, but do they prevent death? Or do they prevent serious consequences?" She and her colleagues in the Cochrane Collaboration have helped to spark much-needed public conversation in the flood of pinkified breast cancer awareness campaigning every October.

The evidence around mammography is accumulating. The picture has changed from one in which mammography screening was believed to be an enormous lifesaver to one of a program in which about 2,000 women over age 50 would need to be screened for ten years to prevent only *one* from dying from breast cancer. At the same time, ten completely healthy women out of those 2,000 would be diagnosed and treated unnecessarily. These unnecessary treatments can be harmful.

Even as the world gets a clearer understanding of the limitations of mammography, there are those, such as Peter Gøtzsche, a Danish researcher and the director of the Nordic Cochrane Centre, who think we need to go further.[11]

He has been researching mammography for more than a decade, and at first his suggestions regarding the overdiagnosis of breast cancer were considered wildly over the top. But now they have gone mainstream.

Reduce Risk by Halting Screening

Gøtzsche's 2011 article in the *Canadian Medical Association Journal*[12] contains an assertion that some find impossible to believe; provocative even, although it is likely true: "The best method we have to reduce the risk of breast cancer is to stop the screening program." For such a strong assertion, of course, careful collection of evidence is necessary. He and his colleagues have scrupulously gathered it.

While the controversy has been building for years, Gøtzsche's article was, up to that point, perhaps the strongest argument against mammography screening ever seen in the pages of a prominent medical journal. In the commentary, Gøtzsche says that the key problem with breast cancer screening is overdiagnosis – which is to say, sometimes what might appear to be a deadly cancer isn't.

Slight lesions in the milk ducts in a woman's breasts may look like cancer. When discovered on a mammogram, a cascade begins: depression, anxiety, biopsies, surgery, radiotherapy and drugs – even if the lesions would never have gone on to hurt the woman.

Gøtzsche was once called the "Cochrane Collaboration's Doberman."[13] That's a reasonably accurate moniker, especially in contrast to the packs braying the benefits of mammography every October. Gøtzsche is a dog that likes to bark – and occasionally bite.

He never really intended to become a world authority on the evidence behind mammography. "I didn't have any interest in mammography screening and I didn't know anything about it until I was asked in 1999 to review the trials for the Danish Board of Health. This was because there had been a Swedish study that couldn't see any effect of mammography screening in Sweden, which was one of the first countries to start mammography screening. So we did this report in just four weeks and concluded that it was doubtful whether it worked and it might do more harm than good." That finding got his attention, especially at a time when breast cancer screening programs were ramping up all over the world.

Gøtzsche continues: "Then we were asked to do a more detailed review ... and we even got funded for doing a Cochrane review." For him, "the interesting thing is that what we still say about mammography screening today, 12 years later, but with much more data, is that the benefit is small – much [smaller] than what has been claimed – and there is a lot of over-diagnosis." He is unequivocal in his thoughts about mammography, saying it "converts a lot of healthy women into cancer patients unnecessarily."

Gøtzsche's willingness to challenge the authorities of his day and to demand better evidence for screening might suggest that asking hard questions about any healthcare procedure can be beneficial to patients. Accordingly, he is also highly critical of the PSA test, a blood screening test to determine the likelihood that a man has prostate cancer.

The PSA test has been widely promoted for many years, but systematic reviews clearly document evidence for risk of harm because of over-diagnosis. In 2012, the United States Preventive Services Task Force, a large independent body that advises on screening, said that the PSA test is no longer recommended for healthy men in the United States.[14] Canada came to the same conclusion in 2014. Gøtzsche is pretty firm about what that means for him: "No one comes near my prostate."

Why? Gøtzsche says, "The harms are so tremendous, and it's a biological fact that people at my age have cancer in their body and that cancer fortunately is usually very benign. It disappears again. The body takes care of it or it grows so slowly it doesn't matter. I believe this is what has made mammography screening so controversial."

He stresses that looking for harms from over-diagnosis and over-treatment is important because other research might discount those things. He said, "We were actually the first ones, I think, who demonstrated it in an analysis back in 2000, and it has been pretty much ignored by screening advocates ever since."

Over the years, he says, other research has used different statistical models claiming that the over-diagnosis rate was pretty small. He said, "There have been a lot of battles and there are lots of vested interests here, which people don't usually think about. There are lots of careers … lots of money involved, and there are, of course, the beliefs that we do something good."

Gøtzsche's reviews on screening's limitations have found that the "level of over-diagnosis is about 50 per cent in those countries that have organized screening programs." He didn't shy away from the controversy in his editorial in the *CMAJ*, saying, "If screening had been a drug, it would have been withdrawn from the market." The article ends with a challenge wrapped up in a provocative question: "Which country will be first to stop mammography screening?"

This is an important question on two fronts: the benefit/harm implications for patients and the financial costs to patients and national health systems. The sheer financial impact of mammography is undeniable. In the USA, it is estimated that biennial mammography screening might cost US$4 billion a year. But the real expense is in all that happens afterwards. The price tag for all the follow-up biopsies triggered by false-positive mammograms has been estimated at between US$14 billion and $70 billion annually.[15]

The impact, then, of Gøtzsche's reviews of mammography could be huge to the sustainability of health systems. As countries including China, Brazil and India continue to develop, the growing middle classes around the world will start demanding access to medical advances that people in the industrialized world have had for years, including programs such as mammography screening. Gøtzsche's Cochrane reviews have the potential to affect policy decisions on breast cancer screening for hundreds of millions of women at a time when there is a massive push to offer these technologies to women in developing countries.

Gøtzsche is one of the Collaboration's most outspoken dissidents, but he's not the only one. There are tens of thousands of people involved in the Cochrane Collaboration all over the globe, from many different walks of life. They are providers of health care (doctors, nurses, physiotherapists and anesthetists, to name but a few), researchers, scientists, university professors, statisticians, economists and (most importantly) people who need effective health care, such as you and I.

Many of the people in this incredibly diverse group have experienced that "aha" moment and said, "There is a problem here, but maybe I can make a difference."

When I asked Gøtzsche, one of the Collaboration's founding members, why he chose to be involved in creating systematic reviews of healthcare interventions, I thought it was a simple question. He explained that his career trajectory originally would have led him to become a professor of internal medicine. Then the Cochrane Collaboration started. Within four years, Gøtzsche had stopped seeing patients.

The tall, hearty Dane is less fearful of speaking his mind than probably anyone I have yet met – in or outside the Collaboration. He did not hesitate to pinpoint his own "aha" moment: "I realized that, as a doctor, I could treat one patient at a time, but by doing a review with the Collaboration, I could treat tens of thousands of patients at a time."

It's a lesson that members of the Collaboration around the world keep relearning: by collaborating with others, seeking high-quality evidence, critically examining it, and then making it widely available, you can multiply the effects of your effort thousands of times, and perhaps for billions of people.

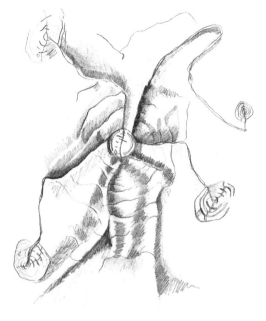

TWO

Iain Chalmers, Archie Cochrane, and the Jibe That Changed Everything

"It changed my life." [16]

— Sir Iain Chalmers

WHO HASN'T experienced things that altered the course of their life? A large tree falls into a stream, and suddenly the water changes direction. Haven't we all had those moments that interrupt life's course and send us off in a different arc?

I have often heard people involved in the Cochrane Collaboration say, "It changed my life." Sometimes, the "it" refers to a chance meeting or a lecture, a conversation, or even a jibe. For many over the last 20 years, the "it" is the Collaboration itself.

Iain Chalmers introduces himself humbly and simply, as "one of the co-founders of the Cochrane Collaboration," as well as "for ten years (1992 to 2002), director of the first Cochrane Centre, here in Oxford."[17]

Know What's Good

When he says, "It changed my life," he's referring to a slim green book written by Archie Cochrane and published in 1972. It is entitled *Effectiveness and Efficiency: Random Reflections on Health Services*[18]. Archie was both a physician and an epidemiologist – someone who studies the patterns and causes and effects of diseases and interventions. His dual interest – in the wellbeing of communities as well as in the care of individuals – does not make him a particularly unique figure, but the words in that book and the sentiment it carried arrived at possibly a seminal time in history. There were some action-oriented people clearly ready to receive them.

People like Iain Chalmers, who think deeply about the basis of health care, are really philosophers at heart – epistemologists to be exact. Epistemologists ask how one can know if something is true. Are there valid ways to distinguish truth from opinion? What measures should we use to distinguish truths from falsehoods? After all, in medicine, if you can't separate what's reliably proven and probably true from what's not proven and possibly false, then you can never be sure if the health care you're providing will help and not harm.

Cochrane's *Effectiveness and Efficiency* became an influential bestseller and clearly had a transformative effect on many people. It asserted that randomized trials are among the least biased ways to identify which health services are likely to do more good than harm.

Some types of research are likely to be more reliable than others, especially ones in which groups of similar patients are randomly allocated to competing treatments, in ways that can reduce bias. Archie may be best known for thinking and writing about randomization, but how he carried out his own research reveals much about his character. To engage in epidemiology, you need a population of patients – the larger the better – and you need a particular disease. The population must have that disease.

As his research population, Archie looked to coal miners in South Wales. He categorized the types of lung disease that coal miners frequently get from breathing coal dust and tracked how dust exposure related to disability. This is the kind of research that takes a lot of time, because it can take many years of exposure to develop disease, as it does for smoking and lung cancer, for example. Good quality epidemiologic research depends on being meticulous, keeping exact records, monitoring closely, and doing whatever it takes to keep in contact with the people in your study so that you can follow up with them.

If you can't maintain contact with the people in the population you are studying, then you won't know how they fared over time – if they improved or got worse because of an intervention – and that would be a tragic loss of meaning and power. Almost the number-one mission in epidemiology is that *you must follow up.* The tragedy of having too many missing people in the course of a trial is that you'll never know what the full jigsaw puzzle is supposed to look like. Missing data are abhorrent to epidemiologic research because their absence compromises the whole picture.

Archie Cochrane was noted for his exceptional follow-up. His studies tracked and re-surveyed miners sometimes 20 or 30 years after the beginning of the study (which nowadays is rare; many studies might last 2 or 3 or 5 years at most). Iain Chalmers wrote that Archie's success in tracking patients followed from his employing disabled miners to help him with the data collection at a time when that job was usually left to professional researchers. This alone might have been his key to such fabulous follow-up rates. After all, if you're a miner, whom do you trust to take down your story accurately: one of your own, or some nerd from the university?

In the introduction to his little green book, Cochrane recalls an incident in the 1930s, when he was a medical student attending a rally in a London suburb. The subject of the demonstration was the establishment of a National Health Service in the UK, and young Archie, an independent thinker who admittedly had difficulty fitting into organizations, chose to scrawl out his own slogan on a banner:

"All effective care must be free."

While he later declared his "adolescent inspiration" a "flop" (he sardonically noted that the one person who read his banner accused him of being a Trotskyite), it captures the heart of his conception of health care. At the time, the world was in a global economic depression. Poverty and unemployment were rife in his country, and he admits that he was "emotionally biased in favour of the idea of an NHS." Even though Cochrane's wealthy Scottish tweed-making family left him with a reasonable inheritance, he was acutely aware of the world's inequalities and wrote that his thoughts were influenced by the "social injustices I saw in the 1930s."[19]

The yearning for a national health service in any nation arises from its collective will and humanity. It is driven by the idea that people deserve equitable access to health care, regardless of their ability to pay for it. But, as Archie Cochrane understood deeply, for universal health care to be a reality, governments would have to use their limited resources wisely to pay for healthcare services that are effective.

One might say that the operative word in Archie Cochrane's youthful slogan is not "free" but "effective." Indeed, the slogan could be re-stated as "All free care must be effective." Anyone designing a healthcare system for all must work hard to determine what can be considered effective.

Yet, how does one determine effectiveness in health care? Do you take advice from experts? What happens when the experts themselves disagree about ways to treat and prevent health problems? Iain Chalmers writes that, as a young doctor, he felt ill-equipped to assess conflicting opinions of senior doctors. In his understated way, Chalmers said that Cochrane's book "introduced me in an evening to the notion that research might be helpful in assessing who was most likely to be right."[20]

Perhaps the most important question that one could draw from Cochrane's book is what one could call "the Cochrane Question":

"How can we have a rational health service if we don't know which of the things being done in it are useful and which are useless or possibly even harmful?"

Randomization and good, methodical record-keeping are important to help determine which therapies are likely to be effective. Archie Cochrane demonstrated, in the desperation of his incarceration in a German prisoner-of-war (POW) camp, that even when no effective care was available, the least that physicians could do was to treat patients with humanity and dignity. Even holding a dying patient in his arms when no medicine or other help was available would pass the test of providing humane and "effective" care.

People Often Get Better on Their Own

Most people would assume that Archie Cochrane must have been a great man. By his own account, he "didn't do too badly." He was an honest and resourceful physician who led groundbreaking work in epidemiology and health services research. He survived grueling conditions in the battlefields of Spain during the Spanish Civil War and in several German POW camps.

Recounting his days as a POW, stuck in a camp at Salonika, Cochrane had virtually nothing with which to treat the illness all around him – typhoid, diphtheria, and jaundice. Here he was, a single doctor with little medicine and surrounded by illness. He once asked the German doctor for more medical help: in particular, more doctors to treat the POWs. The German replied, "Nein. Ärtze sind überflüssig." ("No. Doctors are superfluous.")

Later, he wrote, "I wondered if he was wise or cruel. He was certainly right."[21]

Doctors *are* superfluous? How can that be so? It's probably because of one simple but often-forgotten fact about illness: a good number of patients who get sick also get well on their own, with little or no medical help. Cochrane found that, despite the POWs' dire living conditions, few died.

In a camp of 20,000 prisoners, he expected hundreds to die of diphtheria, as there were no specific medicines for them. Yet, in the six months he was in Salonika, there were only four deaths under his care, three of them by German gunshot wounds. In his characteristic self-deprecating way, he admitted that, "this excellent result had, of course, nothing to do with the therapy they received or my clinical skill." He added that his situation "demonstrated very clearly, on the other hand, the relative unimportance of therapy in comparison with the recuperative power of the human body."

What Cochrane admitted that he most lacked in the POW camps was knowledge on what to do with all the various forms of sickness around him. He would have gladly sacrificed his "freedom for a little knowledge."[22] Since he had neither, he was driven by circumstance to test simple ways to help his fellow inmates. Many of the prisoners were suffering from a form of very painful pitting edema, or swelling above the knees. He had the condition

THE COCHRANE COLLABORATION • 23

himself and wondered what kind of nutritional deficiency could be causing it.

Cochrane recalled the experiment of his own hero, James Lind, a surgeon in Britain's Royal Navy who conducted a simple controlled trial in 1747 to determine the best way to treat scurvy in Royal Navy sailors. Archie Cochrane reasoned that perhaps the prisoners' pitting edema was caused by a vitamin deficiency, so he set up a trial.

He selected 20 prisoners with pitting edema, gave each of them a number, and assigned those with odd numbers to a ward where each of them received two spoonfuls of yeast daily. Those with even numbers went to a ward where each received a tablet of Vitamin C every day. Admitting it was a crude experiment, he still found what worked: The patients on the yeast began to heal. With this answer, he asked the German authorities to supply the camp with yeast to help treat his patients. Surprisingly, they did.

Perhaps doctors might have been merely superfluous, but at the same time, they might also have been harming their patients. Cochrane wrote that his second POW experience, in Elsterhorst, found him in better-equipped conditions but with many prisoners suffering greatly from tuberculosis. It was a desperate situation, and he reported, "there was no real evidence that anything we had to offer had any effect on tuberculosis, and I was afraid that I shortened the lives of some of my friends by unnecessary intervention."

This kind of admission, no doubt, can be the tree that falls into one's stream, causing the course of one's life to change in unexpected ways.

Doctors are trained to save lives; to apply their knowledge and experience as best they can to save their patients. They might take an oath to do no harm, but they must know that any drug with beneficial effects can also have harmful effects. When things line up, with a mixture of luck and science, doctors can save lives and make lives worth living. When they don't, doctors may not only fail to help, but they may also harm their patients. Archie Cochrane demonstrated that when neither luck nor science is on your side, a physician can provide a bit of humanity and dignity, even when it won't change the eventual outcome. After the war, Cochrane started carrying out his research with the Welsh miners and proselytizing about randomization and the importance of properly designed trials to assess the effects of treatments. When there is genuine uncertainty about the effects of a treatment, using it would be considered unethical. He also did something that was perhaps as dangerous as trying to practice medicine in a German POW camp: he challenged his profession to do better.

Cochrane's Jibe

When Iain Chalmers read Archie Cochrane's masterpiece, he said it changed his life, calling *Effectiveness and Efficiency* a "compass in the jungle." It's that one book that he said inspired him to create what would, 20 years later, become the foundation for the international Cochrane Collaboration.

I'd call Chalmers a driven "truth seeker." He knows that people – and even highly intelligent people, the kind that you would find as doctors and medical specialists – can be misled by biases and the play of chance. Because of this, one has to be strenuous – some might say obsessive – in avoiding biases of all stripes, because if physicians are misled, then patients may be harmed.

Chalmers admitted that, after medical school, he wasn't properly equipped to decide what to do when conflicting opinions were presented. Referring to his early experiences in medicine, he said, "I didn't know how to go about judging who was right. My training at medical school hadn't left me with any tools with which to investigate that dilemma."[23]

His exposure to Archie Cochrane's ideas was a lifesaver,

especially the fact that Cochrane "went on to actually indicate where one might start to find the answers." When faced with many opinions, said Chalmers, you have to remember that "not all opinions are equal. Some are supported by mediocre research. Some are based on rigorous research." Randomized trials, for Chalmers, represented a way to navigate around "conflicting and incompatible clinical opinions about how to practice." He began looking for trial reports in his field of interest, obstetrics.

He started in the mid-70s, "right about 1974," said Chalmers, and "I decided we needed to look systematically for these studies because you couldn't at that time find them easily through the bibliographic databases. You had to look for them by hand."

He was also growing interested in the new field of meta-analysis, which he describes as "analyzing similar studies together so that one could start to address the way you can be misled by the play of chance."

As Chalmers and his colleagues were searching in earnest for controlled trials in perinatal medicine, he also outlined how to carry out a systematic review of such trials. Two years later, the World Health Organization and the Department of Health in England began to fund the National Perinatal Epidemiology Unit, in Oxford. Chalmers was asked to direct it. The goal: to assemble a register of controlled trials in perinatal medicine.

When I asked him about this time, he said that his work was gaining momentum, but he pointed to the challenge set forth by Archie Cochrane and his book, which he called "the basis for the Cochrane Collaboration." It was, he said with characteristic modesty, "quite a good challenge for us to actually get on and do something about it."

While Archie Cochrane's slim 1972 book changed the life of Iain Chalmers, his 1979 jibe ended up changing everything. Here is what Iain Chalmers once euphemistically called "Cochrane's Jibe":

"It is surely a great criticism of our profession that we have not organised a critical summary, by specialty or subspecialty, adapted periodically, of all relevant randomised controlled trials."[24]

Chalmers wrote that "a few years after [Cochrane's] death, this [jibe] proved to be the rallying point that led to the creation of the Cochrane Collaboration."[25]

Let me paraphrase Cochrane's jibe: He and his colleagues (doctors, and perhaps all health professionals) deserved to be roundly criticized for not doing something so simple and so necessary, that they should be ashamed of themselves for not doing it: organizing sets of critical summaries of the best evidence of the effects of the various health interventions, and keeping those summaries current.

There was simply no puncturing this astute observation. Even in the debates that followed, the fierce criticisms of evidence-based medicine and the disparagements thrown at the Cochrane Collaboration, no one, as far as I can tell, has come up with anything that effectively counters Archie Cochrane's jibe. The inference of this is that, without high-quality evidence, the basis for the health care being offered to patients remains uncertain.

A jibe is defined as an insulting or mocking remark, a taunt. There are few ways to respond to one: Ignore it, or take the criticism to heart. Maybe Cochrane's jibe wouldn't have had the effect that it did had Cochrane not isolated a specialty that was particularly bad at evidence-based care. But to make his jibe even more piquant, Cochrane picked on Iain Chalmers' specialty, calling obstetrics the "least scientific medical specialty."

From Wooden Spoon to "Real Milestone"

Cochrane awarded obstetrics the "wooden spoon," an award which showed his University of Cambridge roots. At Cambridge, the spoon was typically awarded to the person who scored the lowest exam marks. The term went on in other iterations as the name for the booby prize – the thing you give to someone who finishes last.

When I was a child, getting a wooden spoon meant something different. It was what a parent would use to apply corporal punishment, usually via a child's backside. Getting a whack with a wooden spoon usually had this effect on you: you remembered acutely why you got whacked, and you vowed to yourself not to do that again.

The sentiment that obstetric medicine wasn't very scientific – and deserved to be whacked with a wooden spoon – was something that Chalmers would likely have agreed with, even in his early days practising obstetrics in Cardiff.

Jan Chalmers, Iain's wife and a nurse, recalled, "I think … this [all] started in the maternity hospital.[26] Women were coming to the clinics and they were all being weighed every time they came. They were all having their blood pressure taken every time they came. And each woman that came had to undergo the program of the doctor she was seeing. And [Iain] suddenly felt all these consultants are giving these women different regimes. Which one is right? They can't all be right! I mean they can't all be wrong either. So that was when he became interested in why we subject people to all these different treatments." This experience, she said, stoked Chalmers' interest in the field of determining what was most likely right.

Iain Chalmers said that Archie Cochrane was "particularly annoyed that there had been quite massive changes in obstetrics and gynecology policy based on very threadbare evidence." That was also reflected in what he was seeing in the way pregnancy and childbirth were becoming increasingly medicalized. He said that there was a growing "public unease about the nature of the maternity services in this country, with high intervention rates, growing cesarean section use, and induction of labor." The idea of "daylight deliveries" was taking hold, where, in Chalmers' words, "everyone could do a nine-to-five job as long as they induced labor at 9:00 a.m. and could finish their day at 5:00."

Wooden spoon indeed.

Authority Challenged Over Ludicrous, Arbitrary Care

Another researcher who was perhaps even more appalled at the state of maternity care, and who saw an urgent need for change, was Murray Enkin, a Canadian obstetrician. When Enkin discovered Chalmers' work, it was as if a tree had fallen into his creek and changed the course of his life. He told me that he had been railing against the barbaric practices of obstetric care (largely unsuccessfully) for nearly 30 years when he met Chalmers.

Murray Enkin is almost 20 years older than Chalmers. Luckily for me, he and his wife Eleanor live near my house in Victoria, Canada. I spoke with him in April of 2012, as he was unpacking boxes after his recent move from Toronto. I asked him what it was like doing obstetric care 60 years ago (he graduated from University of Toronto medical school in 1947). He got a little riled when he spoke of it.

He told me, "Unless you were actually there, you can't really believe what obstetrics was like. A woman went to the hospital to have her baby, and as soon as she entered the hospital, she ceased to be a woman. She became a patient, put into a wheelchair, separated from her clothes, separated from any of her support people, her husband, or anything else, wheeled upstairs, and almost immediately given a narcotic – maybe morphine, or pethidine, or perhaps the most popular was heroin, and a barbiturate sedative, or paraldehyde and hyoscine as an amnesic. And she became screaming and demented. I mean, the sounds in a labor room were very similar to what you would expect in a torture chamber. And when she became fully dilated, she was put to sleep with chloroform or ether, and the baby was pulled out. And we had all sorts of ways of resuscitating babies with hot and cold baths to stimulate the breathing and so on."[27]

He waved his hand in a manner of a man who has seen it all. "I mean, that was the whole thing of it. And you couldn't question it because that's the way it was done. It just seemed so terribly wrong to me."

Enkin remembers the day he met Iain Chalmers. He was at a Maternity Center Association conference in 1978. He said, "I think it was their 60th anniversary, and they had a conference in Harriman, New York – an invitational conference. And they were almost all Americans there. As far as I can recall, I was the only Canadian invited."

One of the first lectures was by this British guy I'd never heard of named Iain Chalmers. And I was just absolutely wowed. He was bringing out ideas that resonated so much with what I believed, especially the uselessness of some of the obstetric routines of the day. And he had a book with him called *Benefits and Hazards of the New Obstetrics*.[28] It was hot off the press. And I said, 'Can I … read it?' And he said, 'Well, I got the only copy that's available. You can have it for tonight.'"

Enkin continued, growing more animated as he told his tale: "So, I stayed up all night reading it, and in the morning I was totally hooked." The next morning, he phoned his wife, Eleanor, in Hamilton, and said to her, "This is the guy I've gotta learn from." He laughed when he recalled what he said next: "I said, if I can get him to take me for a sabbatical, would you go to Oxford?"

Of course, Eleanor said yes, and so Enkin asked Chalmers if he could go to Oxford to work with him. Chalmers thought that was a good idea, so Eleanor and Murray headed to Oxford.

Enkin said he's always been a bit of an iconoclast: "I started objecting to obstetric practices when I was still a medical student. And by the early '50s, I was already very dogmatic about it." He added, "I was already 20 years in practice and still pushing the same tired horse. And all of a sudden, the concept of randomized trials and evidence came out."

He said that the science, specifically proper trials, needed to be employed to challenge the "ludicrous" authority and arbitrary nature of maternity care. "It was very good for beating down authority. I mean, for instance, all women had to have their pubic hair shaved when they had a baby? The trials showed that this increased infection. Enemas were another example. You had to give the woman an enema? It was crazy. But you had to do a trial showing that those things didn't work."

Armchair historians often trivialize history by pointing to single events that change its course. History's more complicated than that. But in this light, even though Chalmers and others in many fields were doing what Cochrane said needed to be done, Cochrane's jibe might have altered the course of history. It certainly fired up the motivation of Chalmers, Enkin, and colleagues to lay the groundwork to come up with an answer to it.

Rooting Out Bias the Hard Way

It wasn't only Chalmers' field of perinatal medicine that was influenced by Cochrane's jibe. Other fields, particularly those focusing on specific treatments for diseases such as cancer and heart disease, were also inspired by the idea of creating critical summaries. The difference was a matter of scale.

Even though other researchers at the time were trying to do systematic reviews of specific treatments, Chalmers and his colleagues went a step further: "We were completely mad and ambitious, and decided we ought to try and do it for all of our specialty, for the whole of obstetrics."

Enkin recalls those early pre-computer days when they were searching through the literature. He said that Eleanor did a lot of the work. "You would put a reference on an index card – we used four-by-six cards – and you filed the cards and then sorted them. And we devised a classification scheme."

He explains how they tried to use MEDLINE (a database produced by the National Institutes of Health in the USA that contains journal abstracts and citations from the world's store of biomedical literature), but they found "the classification was completely inadequate."

So, he explained, "We developed a new classification for perinatal literature based on three things: the disease, the intervention, and the outcome." After developing this classification scheme, they went forth to classify all of the literature they could find. It was all done by hand.

There was a small corps of people doing this work but Chalmers, ever the networker, got a lot of help. He said, "Over the subsequent ten years, I suppose, we assembled a team of about 100 people from around the world to get to grips with finding the relevant studies, taking a systematic approach to analyzing and systematizing the results, to come up with whatever seemed to be the most reliable answer for a particular question."

One of those drawn in around this time was Kay Dickersin. She was a PhD student in epidemiology, in her thirties with two young children, when her husband decided to go to medical school. This meant moving the family to Boston, and Dickersin going to work. She found out that the renowned Tom Chalmers (see Chapter 4) was on sabbatical at the Harvard School of Public Health, so she went to see him to find out if there was something she could work on with him.

Tom Chalmers was teaching a course on meta-analysis, and his students in the course included John Simes and Alessandro Liberati, who ended up working with the Cochrane Collaboration. To make an interesting story exceedingly short, Dickersin was put in touch with Iain Chalmers to help develop a trials registry in the perinatal area, which was being expanded to include unpublished and ongoing trials. She went to Oxford to write a grant proposal (which became her thesis) and the Project on Publication Bias in Clinical Trials was where Tom Chalmers, Iain Chalmers, and Kay Dickersin all started working together. Between about 1979 and 1989 was a decade of hard-slogging work, mining through journals and digging through stacks of literature to find trials. This involved an impressive worldwide survey of more than 40,000 obstetricians, pediatricians, midwives, and neonatal nurses around the world to try to uncover unpublished studies.

As Iain Chalmers noted, it was essential to scour for research that didn't make it into the medical literature, because if the unpublished studies weren't included in the overall body of research that had been conducted, then "we would almost certainly be misleading ourselves."

What Iain Chalmers described as "two thunderous great books," the two-volume *Effective Care in Pregnancy and Childbirth*[29], co-authored with Murray Enkin and Marc Keirse, came out of the work done during that period. The essence of this enormous effort was also encapsulated into a smaller paperback for women because, Iain said, "we wanted them to have access to the results of our research."

Iain and Tom Chalmers were early proponents of trial registries. Iain agreed that it seemed mad to have to survey thousands of people to find appropriate research. He said that the right way to deal with the problem is by "registration of controlled trials, prospectively, at inception, before their results are known." It's a theme that Iain Chalmers and others in the Collaboration have kept alive to this day.

Another problem that Iain and others realized early on was that, whenever you publish something on paper, you might as well write it on papyrus, because it soon becomes an out-of-date relic. Luckily, the personal-computer revolution was starting to take off at that time. Publishing electronically became an obvious and serendipitous solution to the problem of keeping things up to date.

Iain Chalmers' group started publishing electronically in 1988, in what was initially known as the *Oxford Database of Perinatal Trials*[30] and continues to be available as part of the Pregnancy and Childbirth module of the Cochrane Collaboration.

Challenging Authority with Good Data

As a table typically has four legs, it might be said that the Cochrane Collaboration rests on a four-legged foundation.

The American Dan Fox was the long-time president (1990 to 2007) of the Milbank Memorial Fund, a nonprofit group that tries to marry good research with health policy and practice. He has been an enthusiastic cheerleader for bringing evidence to the rescue of health policymaking in the USA and around the world. In summing up the early work of Iain Chalmers and colleagues, he wrote that four interrelated publications in obstetrics between 1988 and 1992 have been critical in influencing both health policy and the way medicine is practiced:

1. *The Oxford Database of Perinatal Trials* (ODPT)
2. *Effective Care in Pregnancy and Childbirth* (ECPC)
3. *A Guide to Effective Care in Pregnancy and Childbirth* (GECPC)[31]
4. *Effective Care of the Newborn Infant* (ECNI)[32]

In Fox's estimation, "These publications applied and advanced methods that had a substantial history in the medical, biological, physical and social sciences." He concluded that this four-legged table showed that it was feasible to organize and sustain "programs to conduct systematic reviews across an entire field of health care."[33]

These four works not only proved the concept, but, Fox writes, "the publications also influenced subsequent advances in the methodology of systematic reviews and contributed to their proliferation, in large measure, but not entirely, because their editors and many of the authors participated in organizing and developing the Cochrane Collaboration."[34]

These four accomplishments also did something else. They made it acceptable to question the bases of healthcare decisions. Creating an evidence-based standard for one area of medical care now seems quaint, but you can't underestimate how challenging this change in attitude would have been for practitioners and patients as these trials databases and systematic reviews were made public. In the words of Jini Hetherington, "I think for a busy clinician who has been working for years dishing out treatment of one sort or another, completely unchallenged ... and then someone comes along and says, 'Hang on a minute. How do you know that what you're doing isn't doing more harm than good?' That can feel like quite an affront." [35]

Iain Chalmers calls Hetherington his "closest and longest standing collaborator" and when I interviewed her she was a boundless source of information, inspiration and plain old gossip, having been with the Collaboration before it was even a glint in Iain Chalmers' eye. She has an uncanny, but extremely diplomatic way to "tell it like it is" and some would say she's been a good part of the glue that has kept the Collaboration functioning for 20 years.

Beyond all the accolades and praise for the accomplishments of Iain Chalmers and his colleagues, maybe Hetherington's words sum up the main thing that the Collaboration has planted in the ordinary person: that when it comes to their own health care a person needs the freedom and the opportunity to ask questions and to question answers. And at the very least, to say, in her words, "Hang on a minute."

Perhaps one might say that the four products mentioned above were together a package. It was all part of Iain Chalmers' response to Cochrane's jibe.

The package was rock-solid proof that what Archie Cochrane suggested needed to be done, could be done. With this triumph, Iain Chalmers said, in his understated way, that it was now "possible to conceptualize what the Cochrane Collaboration might do if there were sufficient support for it."

A Real Milestone

For Chalmers and his colleagues who had once felt the sting of the wooden spoon, their decade of hard work was rewarded with some kind words from Archie Cochrane himself. He lived long enough to see this response to his jibe, in the area that he had once judged to be the least evidence-based.

Archie wrote in the foreword to the 1,500-page, two-volume *Effective Care in Pregnancy and Childbirth* that it represented "a real milestone in the history of randomized trials and in the evaluation of care."[36]

Yet in praising this enormous accomplishment, Cochrane clearly hadn't run out of jibes. He had one more. He said that other specialties should copy what Iain and his colleagues had done.

Archie Cochrane died in 1988, never to see the launch of the organization that now bears his name or the international collaboration it has become. His name was a natural choice for a centre; natural for what Archie stood for, but also resonant, so that every time you hear the name, you might be reminded of his jibe.

The name might be a mild reminder that the job is not yet finished.

New Research Often Premature

Billions of dollars are currently spent around the world on medical research, but the investments in systematic reviews are still paltry by comparison. Doing a systematic review might not seem sexy – certainly not as exciting as discovering a new drug or a chemical pathway or a gene that determines a patient's risk of developing a disease. It is dogged work, done largely in obscurity, and for few accolades.

However, a systematic review can provide exceptional value, especially when you "compare it to doing another primary study, or another controlled trial," says Iain Chalmers. In his opinion, "They are the right way to spend your money if you need to find out whether or not there's a need for a further trial to address particular questions." He maintains that it's a "scandal currently that people aren't systemically doing an assessment of what's known already before embarking on new research."

Undoubtedly, Chalmers' work and the work of the Cochrane Collaboration have helped to put systematic reviews on the map. The stream doesn't flow the way it used to, and the tree that fell into it has altered the course, taking us all in a new direction. There is no going back from this.

Archie Cochrane's book changed Iain Chalmers' life, and Cochrane's jibe changed our understanding of what is possible.

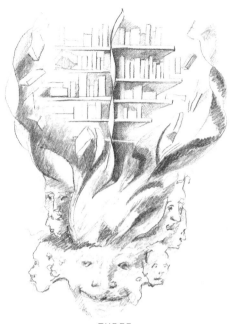

THREE

An Unusual Library:
for Knowledge-based Health Care

*"Like all great ideas, it's so simple and obvious
that it just had to be done."*

— Muir Gray

DR. MUIR GRAY was about to be eaten by a pack of wild dogs and he felt nervous. He was driving his car to High Wycombe, England, to an evening meeting of the British Medical Association, the main lobby group for British physicians – not an organization to be trifled with. Before the group was a debate about this relatively new thing called "evidence-based medicine." *The Lancet* had recently published[37] a hostile editorial, the thrust of which could be summed up, "Who do these people in Oxford think they are?"

Gray wondered how he had got himself into a jam like that, so he did what any sane person would do. He called Iain Chalmers. He said, "Iain, I'm just on my way to Wycombe, and their proposition is, 'This house deplores evidence-based medicine.' It's gonna be me against 100 dogs. What should I say?"

Gray got what he needed.[38] He went into the hall and laid out his opening line: "We'll debate. But our principle is [that] when patients campaign against evidence-based medicine, then we'll listen."

The room went dead. Silence.

"Game over," he said to me, pausing for effect. And then he laughed. "Knocked 'em dead."

Muir Gray has a wild mane of gray hair that shakes when he laughs, which he does often. He's a consummate storyteller, with enough truths peeking out from behind his jests to rivet any listener. He says that he was put on this earth to "keep Iain from going mad,"[39] but he is also the angel investor who helped get the Cochrane Centre, and later the Collaboration, on its feet.

Gray's a physician, an academic, and a bureaucrat, but he doesn't seem to emit the befuddling jargon common to those trades. He says, "I'm more like an engineer. So Iain was the producer of this stuff, but then my job was to think how it influenced what happened in the field."

If you called him the midwife who happened to be there when Iain Chalmers and colleagues were giving birth to the Cochrane Collaboration, he'd credit Chalmers for all the pushing; all the hard work.

In the early 1990s, when the concept of systematic reviews of evidence was starting to gain some traction, Iain Chalmers, Dave Sackett and Muir Gray were often out in the community, making links with physicians, research funders and health policy makers.

After all, they had an important story to tell. If the funders of the health services didn't understand why systematic evidence was important, why would they fund it? Gray and his colleagues needed to keep making the case to health bureaucrats as to why what they were doing was the right thing to do. Not only were they creating systematic reviews, but also making them available to all.

Gray has had a varied career, directing research and development for a number of health authorities in the UK as well as serving as director of the UK National Screening Committee. In 2005, he became Sir Muir Gray, credited for developing screening programs and creating the National Library for Health. His accomplishments are many, but the biggest contribution to Iain Chalmers and the launch of the Cochrane Collaboration might have been his understanding of the inner workings of the National Health Service.

He maintains that there have been two types of changes brought about because of the Cochrane Collaboration: "The overt and the covert. The overt is obviously the creation of the database [of systematic reviews]."

He ladles out some historical context to back up his words: "When we started, there was a study done by... Carol Lefebvre and [other] people here. And I think there were 13,148 trials you could find in MEDLINE when we started." [MEDLINE is a database of journal citations and abstracts from the world's store of biomedical literature.]

"When we went out, and I was in charge of the Cochrane Surgical Trials program at the time, we were doing things like going to old people's clubs in Oxford. We'd describe what a randomized controlled trial was, and even get them to design one, and [we'd] then recruit these retired people to go into libraries and look through every journal. You know, the handsearching." Handsearching is what it sounds like – without a database. You'd have to go to the stacks in a library, open the journals, look at the tables of contents, and find the articles of interest. It is laborious, time-consuming, and very inefficient compared to doing a key-word search of a database to find only those articles that match various search terms.

He continues: "Within about a year, I think we'd found 400,000 trials that had been in MEDLINE but had not been in-dexed." The waste was enormous. He adds, "There was the equivalent of billions of dollars' worth of research that you couldn't find. So the best searcher in the world could only find 13,148 trials when there were probably at that time 350,000 to 400,000 trials in MEDLINE – but just unfindable."

The systematic reviews and sorting of research into databases where one could find the reviews were, in Gray's estimation, the *overt* changes brought about by the Cochrane Collaboration.

The *covert* was the cultural change. He says, "The culture change has been the important thing. To me, a health service – it's got the people and then the organization – and the organization has got a structure, systems and culture. The culture is the key. So the culture was changed as a result of Cochrane."

He adds, "Toyota's had a big influence on me," and recalls once reading a speech by the president of Toyota. What struck him was that its president said that Toyota is a 'knowledge business.' Muir says, "Just when you thought it was a car business, 'No, we're a knowledge business. It's knowledge that we use. That's our core business.' So, you know, health care's a knowledge business. It's not a technology business or a chemical business. It's a knowledge business – knowledge between individuals, and knowledge managed for populations. So, we're now, I think, seeing knowledge as the resource. It's knowledge-based health care."

A Bit of Science, a Bit of Luck

Gray recalls the first time Iain Chalmers explained his national work in perinatal medicine, where Chalmers and his colleagues were trying to collect as much evidence as possible on interventions in pregnancy and childbirth. After Chalmers had told Gray about the mind-boggling amount of work his team had done, writing to thousands of obstetricians worldwide looking for unpublished trials, Gray says that Chalmers' advice was simple: "Don't ever do that." He paused, then added, "Don't ever do it. This was before the internet."

Many of today's modern institutions, including banking, shopping, connecting, finding love and avoiding death, have found a home online. It's increasingly hard to explain to young people who have grown up with the internet what life was like; how we shopped, interacted, or collaborated before it existed.

Among the world's great libraries, the *Cochrane Library* might be the most remarkable one that never really had any bricks and mortar. The Collaboration's literature is organized, arranged, and systematically stored in electronic and web-based forms. Its existence without computers and the internet would be unthinkable.

Pre-internet research was many things. Particularly, it was more strenuous. When it came to gathering medical literature, summarizing it, making it meaningful, and then distributing it around the world, it was really mostly about paper. Once you had a meaningful product printed on paper, you had to deliver it to the people who needed it. Printed information was fixed; it started growing stale as the ink was drying. In an increasingly web-enabled world, text is not so fixed. Updates, changes, revisions, and renewals are all intrinsic to the medium. Part of the message, too.

Gray speaks almost elegiacally about the early days: "We needed a bit of science and a bit of luck" to get the Collaboration off the ground. "The internet," he says, "was our little piece of luck."

By the mid-1980s, the idea of images flying around the world, almost for free, was slowly going from unthinkable to remotely possible. Iain Chalmers remembers the images, specifically the forest plot graphs (or "blobograms") that were emerging from the systematic reviews and meta-analyses of specific obstetric treatments that he and his colleagues had been collecting.

Forest plot graphs present a picture of a meta-analysis. The studies are represented by horizontal lines of varying widths, along which the effectiveness of each is plotted. (The present-day logo of the Cochrane Collaboration is a stylized forest plot.) In obstetrics, for instance, these images showed which treatments worked best to stop the uterus from contracting prematurely, or which drugs worked best for women who were expected to give birth to a premature infant. The availability of these images could save lives.

For those putting together meta-analyses, there was a certain clarity in such pictures, a certain aesthetic appeal. Chalmers told me, "What was really beautiful about these plots, these meta-analyses plots, is that they made clear why people had been misled, depending on which study they happened to have bumped into. Some of them were statistically significantly positive; others weren't. But when you looked at them all together, there was this signal coming out which showed that, in general, the results fell on this side or other of the boundary."

Systematic reviews accessible anywhere in the world – most conveniently, accessibly, and efficiently via the internet – could really bring evidence-based medicine to the very clinics and hospitals attended daily by patients and doctors. The emergent availability of forest plots to anyone needing to study them anywhere exemplified this. The nascence of the internet came to be integral to the nascent Collaboration.

"I've Had an Idea"
Fast forward about six years.

The county of Oxfordshire is part of the flat floodplains of the Thames. Quintessential English countryside, it comprises meandering rivers lined with walking paths and willow trees and medieval-looking masonry bridges.

It was in this lush countryside, along Wolvercote Mill Stream, just north of Oxford, that Chalmers walked one spring morning in 1991. He and his colleagues had recently completed the near-decade-long task of putting together the massive two-volume *Effective Care in Pregnancy and Childbirth*, as well as the *Oxford Database of Perinatal Trials*. Both were attracting attention in the UK and abroad.

Among those paying attention was Dr. Michael Peckham, the newly appointed founding director of the NHS Research and Development Programme in the Department of Health. Peckham supported Chalmers' proposal to establish a centre focusing on evidence-based medicine. He expected that it would take the lessons and methods learned in perinatal research during the previous decade and apply them to other healthcare areas.

Chalmers' colleagues went to look at some offices in Middle Way, in a plain, three-story red-brick building that had originally been Oliver and Gurden's cake factory. Chalmers liked this building as a location for the Cochrane Centre, but he had a problem, which he confided to Gray: The centre didn't have enough money for the rent.

Gray had a regional budget, so he told Chalmers not to worry: "Well, we'll fund the rent. I'll pay the rent." How much was needed to lease? Chalmers wanted more than one floor, and told Gray, "I want the room downstairs. I want to store paper copies of all the randomized controlled trials." Muir, ever the engineer, wondered, "Will the floor hold them?" But that question didn't have to be answered, because "the internet came along."

Gray says that the Cochrane Centre (and, later, the Cochrane Collaboration) could not have existed without technology – specifically, technologies facilitating the ability to collect, store, share, and distribute electronic information. Starting the Cochrane

Centre took a ton of work by a whole team of dedicated volunteers and staff, but no one was busier than Chalmers. Gray points to where Chalmers' office was back then and says, "For two years, I think, Iain was in here every day, every night. When I used to pass at night, going home from London or whatever, the lights were on here. So goodness knows how many hours he worked."

Gray recalls how, not long after the Cochrane Centre was established in 1992, Chalmers called him one Saturday morning and said, "Come in and see me."

Gray described what Chalmers said when he arrived: "'I've had an idea. We need a Cochrane Collaboration.' And the good news is, he said, 'The logo. The same logo will do: CC.' So, he said, 'There won't be any expense.'"

Then came another stroke of luck. The head of the Swedish Council on Health Technology Assessment had read an editorial by Kay Dickersin, Iain Chalmers and Tom Chalmers in the *BMJ* in the fall of 1992[40] ("Getting to Grips with Archie Cochrane's Agenda"). The Council called up Iain Chalmers out of the blue and said, "We'd like to give you 25,000 pounds a year for three years." When asked what they wanted Chalmers to use it for, they said "Anything you'd like. We think what you're doing is important and we think that it would be a very good idea for us to invest in it and help to make it happen." Iain Chalmers said this was terribly helpful. The money funded the Steering Group's travel costs to meet in Hamilton. More important, it provided the international boost that this fledgling organization needed.

Building Databases and Virtual Libraries

Mark Starr was an experimental psychologist living in Vancouver, Canada when his wife, Lesley, was headhunted to be the head of midwifery in Oxfordshire, England. She had been responsible for helping to set up the provision of midwifery in British Columbia. Starr laughed and shrugged when I asked him what he thought of pulling up stakes and moving to Oxford. He said, "I just sort of came along for the ride."

As an experimental psychologist, Starr understood statistics. He was old-school enough to remember doing statistical analysis using punch cards and running them through a humongous mainframe computer. Also, "Meta-analysis came out of psychology, so I was already familiar with it when I ran into Iain."

As Starr got to know Iain Chalmers through Lesley, because of her involvement in the pregnancy and childbirth field, he began to understand what Chalmers was doing. One day, he announced in his nonchalant way, "I could put a nice front end on this" as if writing the code, fixing the bugs, and creating the graphics to express sophisticated meta-analyses were all easy.

Starr told me that he really loved those early days with Chalmers and his colleagues: "It was a fun fit. I thought I'd be here for a year or two, and then we'd move back to Vancouver. It was in the late '80s and it just was fun; something to do."

He said that Oxford University Press was supporting the creation of the "big books" (the two-volume *Effective Care in Pregnancy and Childbirth*) and that "They actually paid me to generate all the graphs in those books, so they wouldn't have to lay them out individually. All of a sudden, the technical side became a money-making opportunity, and I found I could live off it." Initially, he worked alongside Malcolm Newdick, whose company Update Software was doing all the programming necessary. Then Malcolm went off to work for Save the Children in Mozambique, leaving Starr and Update Software.

Starr was inspired by the challenge and the stimulation of working alongside Iain Chalmers, whom he described as "a very hands-on sort of person." Many a weekend, particularly a Sunday afternoon, if you dropped by Chalmers' office, you would have found Chalmers and Starr trying to wrap their heads around a particularly tough problem. By all accounts, Starr was a can-do

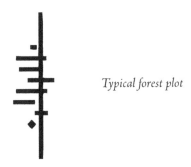

Typical forest plot

sort of programmer. He really wanted to understand what was needed, and his job was to meet those needs with code that would work.

Starr recalled one of the programming tricks that he needed to perfect in the creation of forest plots: "The trick was [that] you could add new studies and then the graph would be redrawn. You could fill in any data, and it would redraw itself and reinterpret itself," he said, adding, "It was one of the first apps, probably. The statisticians have got hold of it and have since made it more complicated, but we were simple in those days."

Starr never did return to Vancouver. He and his wife settled permanently in Oxford. "Things just sort of took off," he said.

Iain Chalmers wrote, "Malcolm Newdick and Mark Starr did the programming necessary to assemble and display all the hundreds of analyses being prepared for the books. At the end of 1988, these were published electronically, together with structured abstracts, and then regularly updated in an electronic journal called the *Oxford Database of Perinatal Trials (ODPT)*, which also contained the register of controlled trials we had assembled. Under Mark Starr's guidance, *ODPT* evolved first into the *Cochrane Pregnancy and Childbirth Database* and then into the pregnancy and childbirth module of the *Cochrane Database of Systematic Reviews*."[41]

Starr effused when he talked about the people he had the

chance to work with, particularly Doug Altman: "Doug makes the stats and everything seem so commonsense. He made a huge difference in everybody's work with the Collaboration, especially around the idea that you could put everything into these forest plots. Once you understand that, you understand everything."

Starr's company, Update Software, at its height, had 12 employees and managed to rent offices in the same building and on the same floor as the Cochrane Centre. He said that it was a specialized company, and even though it was mostly set up to disseminate the *Cochrane Database of Systematic Reviews*, and later the *Cochrane Library*, it also did work for the World Health Organization and the Department of Health.

One more stroke of luck, or genius, as Starr said, was that "all the information was stored and retrieved with a programming language called XML," a rarity in the early days of electronic publishing. The decision to go with XML was something that he said he'd had to fight for and later defend. In hindsight, Starr was almost prophetic, as XML later turned into the standard for web publishing. "It meant we were able to process a lot of information. We also controlled the authoring system," he said. That authoring system, known as RevMan (short for Review Manager) is an interface that allows people putting together reviews to insert them into the master database.

Because the databases were growing, there was a mounting need to network computers, and the Collaboration needed someone to take care of this. It hired Monica Kjeldstrøm, a 23-year-old, just graduated, Danish computer-systems engineer.

Kjeldstrøm became part of the Cochrane family and loved it from the very beginning. By all accounts, the family loved her, too. Not only was she brilliant in helping to solve the growing organization's computer networking and information management challenges (which were surely daunting); according to Jini Hetherington, she had "this amazing skill of disagreeing in

the most nonconfrontational and charming way." It was a skill
that proved useful as she grew to take on different roles in the
Collaboration, including as a member of the Steering Group.[42]

A few years later, with Chalmers' support, Kjeldstrøm moved
back to Copenhagen to direct the Cochrane Collaboration's information management system (IMS), as part of the staff of
the Nordic Cochrane Centre. In addition to RevMan, the pro-
prietary software used to prepare Cochrane reviews, the IMS
team in Copenhagen manages Archie, the Internet-based server
that stores current and past versions of systematic reviews, contact details for Cochrane contributors, and other organizational
documentation.

Kjeldstrøm described it this way: "RevMan... helps authors
write reviews in a very systematic way. You have to do it the same
way each time. It's a very fixed structure, which has automatic
checks – essentially proving the authors have achieved what they
set out to do." Since it is highly structured, it can also be highly
annoying to authors when the system doesn't permit them to pro-
ceed unless they've completed the required fields and checked all
the boxes. In 2013, RevMan was in its fifth version. By some accounts, it takes a certain perseverance to use. It's perfect for those
who like to be guided by a computer program; perhaps less so for
those who have their own ideas and dislike constraints.

After having worked in and played a large number of roles
in the Collaboration for nearly 18 years, Kjeldstrøm was ready
for a new act. She applied for a job as the head of Information
Technology at the Royal Danish Theatre.[43] When she applied for
that job, of course they asked her how her previous experience
would prepare her for this new role. She laughed as she recalled
telling the interviewers that her work with the Collaboration was
good training for the theatre. It had given her "lots of experience
working with drama queens."

Names withheld to protect the innocent.

A New Publisher

The Collaboration was ten years old in 2002, and significant events that year showed how the organization was maturing. In March, Finland and Norway made the *Cochrane Library* free to anyone with internet access; England followed suit in April, making it available through the National electronic Library for Health [NeLH]. And that year, the 10th Cochrane Colloquium was held in Stavanger, Norway.

The central discussion in Stavanger was about the future of the electronic home of the Cochrane Collaboration. A tendering process, led by Mike Clarke (then one of the Steering Group's co-chairs) had been held, and a consultant had been hired to advise the Steering Group on its options. A new publisher, John Wiley and Sons Ltd, had been identified.

When it became clear that the leadership had decided to change publishers, the response from Cochrane contributors was emotional. Some approved the move away from Mark Starr's Update Software, saying that the change indicated that the Collaboration was "growing up," becoming more professional, taking things to a higher level. The switch to an internationally recognized publishing house had clear advantages, primarily the opportunity for the Collaboration to establish a more financially sustainable model.

Others felt that it was selling itself to a soulless, profit-driven corporation in exchange for royalties.

Some pointed out that Starr's tiny company was still innovative and nimble enough to try new things in online publishing. Mark had one big advantage: He knew the Collaboration inside and out. He knew the authors and understood their powerful feelings of ownership of the reviews. He knew that they worked doggedly to make those reviews happen and were heavily invested in what they produced.[44]

There was also some uniqueness to the products. Starr said,

"We had specialized databases, such as the renal database and pregnancy [and childbirth] database." He said that he liked the idea of having systematic reviews at the core and also being a bit freer with other things, "letting the review groups add other things: qualitative studies, reviews of reviews. So long as they kept the core as systematic reviews pure, they could create these subsets, [which] could go beyond the dictates of the central Steering Group."

Starr was understandably upset. So were many people who had worked with him over the years, who considered him an integral part of the Cochrane Collaboration, and had witnessed his tireless efforts to build the *Cochrane Library*'s electronic infrastructure. In Chalmers' opinion, "If it hadn't been for Mark Starr, there wouldn't have been a *Cochrane Library*."

Starr doesn't say the decision to go with Wiley was wrong. It was, however, rather upsetting. It was essentially a divorce. The Collaboration lost a valued and longtime member of the family. And like a divorce, with hurt feeling on all sides, it would take some time to heal.

In April, 2003, the Cochrane Collaboration signed a new publishing agreement with Wiley. More than ten years since that decision, Starr looks back on it philosophically. He said that maybe the Cochrane Collaboration had lost some of its early flavor and color – perhaps even the renegade behavior – but that "it was a fun ride while it lasted."

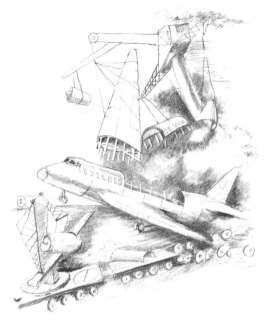

FOUR

Getting Airborne
While Building the Airplane

"So every time I go to the Cochrane Colloquium,
I kind of use Oslo as a control group and say,
'God, look at the difference.'"

— Zarko Alfirevic

Call Me Dave

You could imagine that if Dave Sackett were to write a semi-auto-biographical work of fiction, drawn from the stories of his life and the characters he met along the way, fictionalized to camouflage the innocent, the saints and the bastards, he'd start the book this way: "Call me Dave."

"Call me Dave" might also be Sackett's signature statement. It conveys his unpretentiousness and reflects his dislike for unnecessary formalities.[45]

For a big man, Sackett carried his modesty well. He was big in two senses of the word. First, he was big in the field of evidence-based medicine. Some might call him the godfather of EBM – one of the most acknowledged and ubiquitous early promoters of incorporating good-quality evidence into treatment. He was also big in the physical sense – tall, barrel-chested, and straight-backed; imposing. He had a commanding, steady voice, measured and calm.

Sackett was comfortable adopting and standing behind unpopular viewpoints. He recalled that growing up in the USA during the tumultuous years of the civil rights movement gave him opportunities to ask questions and to be exposed to the language of discrimination. He said, "There was a common phrase in the US as I was growing up about blacks. It would be in the guise of tolerance, where racists would say, "Blacks are okay... in their place." That's a line he pulled out when he reflects on some of the early opposition to evidence-based medicine, especially a particularly nasty *Lancet* editorial titled "*Evidence-based medicine... in its place.*"[46]

He sailed through his medical education, able to memorize the material quickly and flawlessly. Sitting atop his class afforded him some breathing room to ask questions. Later, he found himself in good company with other questioners in the emerging field of clinical epidemiology and evidence-based medicine – questioners such as Archie Cochrane and Tom Chalmers, who were iconoclastic by nature.

One could talk about Sackett's many stellar accomplishments, as he founded one of Canada's best medical schools at the age of thirty-two, founded the Centre for Evidence-Based Medicine in Oxford, was a member of the Canadian Medical Hall of Fame, and was an Order of Canada inductee, among other accolades. He'd say that mentioning these things doesn't advance the narrative of the Cochrane Collaboration.

Sackett's contributions – both overt and covert – definitely have advanced its narrative. Among the overt, he was appointed as the first Chair of the Cochrane Collaboration's Steering Group, which helped to establish the organization's foundations. More covert: his nourishing, through many avenues, of the ideas of evidence-based medicine, as well as his mentorship of the young – bolstering the budding energies and ideas of students and colleagues. That ethos carries on to this day in many others who work under the banner of the Cochrane Collaboration.

The minutes of the Oslo Steering Group meeting in October, 1995 read: "David Sackett outlined his present functions as Chair of the Cochrane Collaboration. He stated his time was spent dealing with conflict resolution, promotion of the Collaboration, and fulfilling the figurehead role." He admitted in his self-deprecating way that he might have been "helpful in getting the Collaboration going," but he was cautious about taking much credit. One thing that emerged in my conversation with him is that he has had many careers in his lifetime.

Whenever he got really good at something, he felt he'd outlived his usefulness and hit the eject button – which is what he did in Oslo. In fact, probably the most telling of Sackett's leadership of the Collaboration is in the circumstances of how it ended. More about this later.

The Inveterate Randomizer

The American physician Tom Chalmers (1917–1995) was one of the twentieth century's great medical thinkers. The New York Academy of Medicine described him as the "acknowledged leader in the design, conduct, and evaluation of clinical trials." Clearly a guy who knew a little bit about trying to find the truth about medical treatments.

I never had a chance to interview Tom Chalmers, yet, I have been able to glean a measure of the man from many who knew him throughout his life, including his daughter,[47] Francie Chalmers. Before his death, Tom Chalmers explained in an interview his own "aha" moment which happened early in his career: "I really did not question the pearls of wisdom from the experts until I got into practice. At some point I said to myself, 'I've killed too many people.'"[48]

This realization drove Chalmers to become a preacher and practitioner of experiments involving random allocation – the best way to determine if health treatments will ultimately help and not hurt patients. In a clinical trial, by randomly allocating participants to treatment and to control groups, and keeping the allocation 'blind' to both participants and researchers (known as a 'double-blind study'), you can eliminate some of the biases that occur.

Tom insisted that our human capacity to fool ourselves knows no bounds, so we must be rigorous about reducing the potential for bias. Whenever there is any uncertainty, the right thing to do is to randomize, for any new medical treatment or surgery; for health authorities deciding to fund new methods of delivering care (such as coronary care units); even for implementing educational programs. He even carried out randomized experiments in his personal life, blinding containers of coffee with his wife (to see if there was any meaningful difference between decaf and regular), and he randomized wine consumed by his family and friends to show how observer bias is alive and well. Even something as simple as a daily commute could be tested through randomization, routinely flipping coins to decide whether to go right or left, then collecting data.[49]

When I talked to Francie Chalmers, Tom's second daughter and a pediatrician living in Washington state, she said, "His mantra was 'Randomize the first patient.' I don't know if it stuck anywhere, but that was his approach. If the choice or answer was not really known, then you had no business making a choice without studying it."

Over the years, Tom Chalmers grew to insist that to best serve humanity, all research studies on similar interventions needed to be methodically gathered together and meta-analyzed for the entire truth they would reveal. Only when this happened and a bullseye emerged from all the relevant studies stacked in a deliberate, logical mosaic, could physicians confidently fulfill their credo: First, do no harm. That mosaic, incidentally, is what is captured in the Cochrane logo.

This inveterate randomizer and proponent of meta-analyses taught, mentored and inspired numerous others in the early days of the Cochrane Collaboration. He attended many of the early meetings and a few of the annual colloquia. He was not involved with the day-to-day operation of the Collaboration, but had a clear influence on many who subsequently played major roles in the group, including Dave Sackett, Brian Haynes, Kay Dickersin, Alessandro Liberati, and others who, Iain Chalmers said, "knew each other's work and obsessions."

In a series of interviews published in the *Canadian Medical Association Journal* in 1996, Tom Chalmers told my mentor and colleague Malcolm Maclure, an epidemiologist at the University of British Columbia, "Patients are way ahead of physicians when it comes to thinking about the advantages of evidence." Iain Chalmers and others in the Cochrane Collaboration echo that sentiment.

Tom said, "People ask me how to improve patient care. I tell them the most important thing for you to do, when a doctor says, 'I'm going to give you this treatment,' is to ask, 'Would you please summarize the evidence in the literature on why this is better than something else for me?'"

Even when faced with a life-threatening diagnosis of prostate cancer, Tom Chalmers went further. He asked the urologist to see if there was a randomized trial in which he could enroll. He did what millions of patients do every year: offer themselves up for the advancement of science. Walk the talk, indeed.

From Academic Science to the Bedside

For some perspective on Tom Chalmers' ideas and the contribution of the Collaboration, I talked to Rory Collins. He is a professor of Medicine and Epidemiology at the University of Oxford, and co-directs the Clinical Trial Service Unit alongside Richard Peto. Peto and Collins are known in the business as mega-trialists: those who plan and conduct large randomized trials, and who have made major contributions to the field of meta-analysis.

Collins went to Oxford in the early 1980s and I asked him how different things looked thirty years later. He told me straightaway: "Cochrane has completely changed people's attitude to evidence."[50]

"First of all," he said, "it has stimulated a very large number of people to get involved in bringing together randomized evidence; to start to understand the value of such evidence across the world."

He said that when Iain Chalmers first spoke to him about the Collaboration, he thought it was "an incredibly ambitious thing to do… an extremely important achievement, especially in bringing together all of the randomized evidence from all areas of medicine so that one knows what's out there."

He adds, "What has changed over the last twenty, thirty years is the recognition that you can usefully combine trials that address the same or similar questions to work out whether or not treatments work. In a sense, it's like the invention of the telescope or a microscope: you could see things that were not otherwise visible by essentially increasing the magnification."

In terms of the Cochrane Collaboration's specific effect on the practice of medicine, Collins thinks it has been in "the sense of getting clinicians to look at all of the evidence, rather than to look at selective parts of the evidence. And I think that that has a lasting impact in terms of how people consider the treatment of patients."

Critical Appraisal Begets Evidence-Based Medicine

Dave Sackett moved to Canada in 1968 to start a new department at a new medical school at McMaster University, Hamilton. At the time, he thought it was just going to be a small department, "Just three of us: me and a statistician and another clinical epidemiologist." The burgeoning new school was organized by the Blood and Cardiovascular Programme and needed a range of scientists including people like Sackett. His department grew tenfold in just a few years. It now includes 150 faculty and similar numbers of staff and graduate students.

Sackett said, "Clinicians across the university began to take some of this epidemiology and biostatistics and use it to assess the literature, because the literature was so vast." He and a few of his protégés, including Brian Haynes and Peter Tugwell (both longstanding members of the Collaboration), developed some "fairly rapid strategies and tactics that clinicians could use to appraise the literature for its validity, but also for its applicability in caring for patients. And we decided to call that 'critical appraisal.'"

Once *critical appraisal* was established, around 1990, Sackett's group thought they needed to take these critical appraisals and begin to "integrate them with patients' values and expectations and come up with better approaches to diagnosis and therapy." Searching for a name for this idea, he said, "a brilliant young colleague, Gordon Guyatt, suggested that we might call it 'evidence-based medicine.' And so that's where all of that began."

Sackett insisted that the Cochrane Collaboration would not have happened without the efforts of Muir Gray who, he said, "had decided that, because what we were doing in evidence-based medicine [at McMaster University] might make a lot of sense in the UK, he [began] to plan for bringing me to Oxford on a full-time basis to set up the Centre for Evidence-Based Medicine."

He liked the idea of going to Oxford, and he met with a small group, including Iain Chalmers, Chris Silagy, Peter Tugwell and Sally Hunt, in the solarium at his house at Irish Lake. He recalled that "they seemed to think that I could be helpful in getting things going. And so it was on that basis that we set up the original Steering Group."

Sackett maintained that, although it might have helped that Muir Gray was out there promoting the Collaboration along with this new thing called evidence-based medicine, "the success of the Cochrane Collaboration right from the start was the unselfish collaboration by people all over the world working together." He spoke with gravity when he said, "It was not some great leadership sort of activity by people like me. It was us enabling those folks; enabling the resources to be made available so that the people who really did the work meant the program could function."

He described his promotion of the young Collaboration as highly indirect: "When I wasn't running the clinical service at the John Radcliffe Hospital, I was almost always on the road, going to district general hospitals all over the UK and then around Europe."

He explained how he introduced evidence on the wards: "I would begin by getting together with the house staff and students, and looking at all the admissions from the previous night," the goal being to show evidence-based medicine in practice at the

bedside with new patients. "Having done that, I would then pro-
ceed from there to give grand rounds again, usually on a clinical
issue where I would demonstrate how, using some of these strategies and tactics [of evidence-based medicine], one might make
a more appropriate diagnosis; one might be able to incorporate
patient values into a therapeutic decision, which might lead to a
better outcome."

A lot of these discussions, which started with the illness of
the patients, came back to the "identification of the necessary
evidence and its integration. And obviously that led then right
into what was going on at the Cochrane Collaboration, because
it would be the really best source of evidence that we could ever
achieve."

He was actively on the road showing people evidence-based
medicine, and he recalled how they would come to the realization that they needed evidence, and there weren't often the proper
studies out there to inform what they were doing. Sackett said:
"People would realize then, at the end of it, all that, 'Gee. This
could work. You've shown how you do it at the bedside. You've
shown how you do it at grand rounds. But then it means we gotta
get the evidence.'"

He added, "By this time, another brilliant colleague of mine,
Brian Haynes, and a group of us had trained a group of research
librarians. We had taught them enough epidemiology and biostatistics so that they took over the reading of journals. Each of
'em read about 50 journals a week. They pulled out every article
about diagnosis, prognosis, therapy, and causation that was sufficiently sound epidemiologically in terms of methods…."

"They then took that stack of articles whose results were likely
to be true, and passed them by a group of folks like us – clinical
epidemiologists, clinicians in various fields with competency in
epidemiology and statistics – and we said, 'Among these articles
that are true, this subset are also clinically relevant and could be

applied right now.' That two-stage process reduced the clinical literature by 98 per cent." And with the leftover 2 per cent, "brilliant Brian Haynes and his team began to put together" a resource which went on to be called the ACP (American College of Physicians) Journal Club, which has grown into being an incredibly popular and solid resource for physicians.

This was what many people putting together Cochrane reviews really wanted to do: take things a step further to produce clear, simple, pragmatic material that was high-quality and relevant to physicians' decision-making (a feat which McMaster is known for, worldwide, and which obsesses people like Gordon Guyatt and Brian Haynes). Sackett said, "Instead of trying to keep up with the journals, which was absolutely impossible, you could, every two months, get a digest in your area of studies, the results of which are true and applicable right now. So, that was one of the sorts of resources we developed."

Not All Fun and Games...
Getting the Cochrane Collaboration and evidence-based medicine to be accepted by the medical culture of Oxford in the early 1990s was not all fun and games. Sackett said, "In many ways it was advantageous to be seen as a Canadian, because so little would be expected of a Canuck in terms of proper manners, and from that it would be excused and it would not be eccentricity. They would simply see you as an amusing rustic," adding in a self-mocking sort of way, "That's the way strange people like me look and behave."

There were a number of important names in the Oxford medical establishment supporting this enterprise created by Iain Chalmers and his colleagues. According to Sackett, "There was this quite good, solid support from a few very senior people, and there was an immediate effect on the young folks." The fact that students warmly embraced evidence-based medicine may partly be attributable to the inner drive of the young to challenge their superiors. Now they had a tool that might make things more interesting. Maybe for some of them, "evidence" became another tool of revolt; a way to 'stick it to the man.'

Looking back on it, Sackett said, "The Cochrane Collaboration was an extraordinarily powerful threat against authority. Individuals who had reputations based upon 'this is the way this disorder must be treated' obviously were terribly threatened by what was going to happen with these young upstarts, and kids, and punks, and even lay people challenging them about what they said must occur in terms of health care."

Sackett admitted that, with his teaching, "We were beginning to equip young people with tools that they could use [to] challenge the professors – not [in] a nasty or flippant sort of way. If a professor was making some authoritarian statement they would say, 'Gee, I would like to learn more about that. Could you point me to the article that would justify this position?' Or, 'Well, professor, I found this particular article that seems to be at variance and contradict what you're saying. Could you take a look at [it with] me and help me understand what was going on?'" He adds, "Other folks were just mad as hell, and were highly resistant and frequently nasty."

Nonetheless, Sackett was surprised how quickly things changed. "When we first went to Oxford, we thought it was probably going to be about a ten-year struggle to get anything going at all. It got picked up so quickly by some of the key senior people, but also so quickly by the young folks, that within about four years we'd accomplished what we thought would take a decade." The ACP Journal Club's sister publication, *Evidence-Based Medicine*, was a huge success, published in six languages, and, "It spread like wildfire."[51]

Friendly Colleagues Stir the Pot

The people at the very core of the Cochrane Collaboration – the Steering Group – were mostly colleagues of Iain Chalmers from the start: Hilda Bastian, Kay Dickersin, Peter Gøtzsche, Brian Haynes, Jos Kleijnen, Alessandro Liberati, Cynthia Mulrow, Andy Oxman, Dave Sackett and Chris Silagy. Many of them had history together. They knew each other's peccadillos and temperaments. And, of course, they were all on a first-name basis.

Hilda Bastian, the first consumer representative on the Steering Group, recalls, "The first few years were very intense in and around the Steering Group, with deep and often bitter conflict around many fundamental issues about the kind of organization it would be." The differences were sometimes political and sometimes philosophical. Some contributors wondered whether the organization would be "highly controlled by a leadership elite." Others wondered if it should be open and democratic. There was a fear in those early days that the Collaboration, which at the time saw itself as a rebel organization, was quickly "succumbing to elitism," in Bastian's words, with the possibility that it could "veer into cultishness."[52]

There was, in her opinion, "a lot of zealotry and 'anointed ones,'" which, she added, were "almost always blokes." The young organization struggled with how long the original leaders could hold their positions. Should it be for life? Should there be periodic elections?

That issue created a crisis for Bastian. She said, "For me, it was either try to change the trajectory or leave. At the first Steering Group meeting, I decided the main way to try to change it was to take on the role of editor of the international newsletter."

In its early days, using a newsletter to communicate with the members of this fledgling organization, who were spread all over the world, seemed a brilliant idea. Bastian became the editor of *Cochrane News* in May, 1995 and held the position until November 1998. As a grassroots community organizer, she felt that the main focus of the newsletter had to be on community building. She pitched its tone to be "deliberately irreverent and folksy," saying she wanted it to exhibit a personality that was encouraging to newcomers. She's unafraid of stirring the pot or even irritating the elites and explained that "irreverence was key to providing an alternative to zealotry and the tendency towards self-righteousness."

Bastian dealt with the political controversies of the Collaboration's early days in a coded way: "in the cartoons – classic newspaper tradition." One cartoon, on page 2 of her first issue, shows a woman standing up in a boardroom full of empty chairs. Reading from her notes, she addresses the room: "Will anyone second the motion that this Committee is too hard to get into?"[53] Bastian describes the cartoon as "not too overt, but setting a tone."

In those early days, pre-internet, when many people didn't yet have e-mail and there wasn't much money for international travel, Bastian felt that the newsletter played "an important role and gave the Collaboration a particular face and personality." It helped to keep people in touch with each other, and in her opinion, "had the potential to influence the culture and play a community-development role."

One sense you get from Bastian is that there has always been a bit of myth-making around the Collaboration. As rigorous as people in the Collaboration are toward science, this rigor doesn't always extend to the Collaboration's own self-image. She thinks that the newsletter was one way for her to continue to be an activist within the organization, and was likely both political and influential, even if people wouldn't admit to that.

Apart from trying to push forward the development of plain

language summaries, Bastian considers the newsletter the most important thing she has done in the Collaboration.

Oslo, Norway, October 4 to 8, 1995

In 1950, the famed Japanese director Akira Kurosawa released the film *Rashomon* to critical acclaim. The film employs a plot device wherein a variety of characters each give their own versions of the same event. It shows, with great art and precision, the fallibility of memory and perception. If you share memories with your friends or siblings of events that happened far in the past, it's likely you've experienced the *Rashomon* effect: in trying to recall an event, it seems as if you'd all experienced something wildly different from each other. The *Rashomon* effect was certainly noticeable as I gathered various recollections of the tumultuous third Cochrane Colloquium in Oslo, Norway in October, 1995.

This meeting occurred when the Collaboration was two years old – barely a toddler. Not quite big enough to run around and set fire to things; still unsure on its feet; cute, but clumsy. You still didn't want to leave sharp objects lying around.

At that point, the output of the Collaboration wasn't much to brag about. There wasn't much in the way of new, completed reviews, but interest in evidence-based medicine and perhaps its highest manifestation – systematic reviews – in many areas of medicine was blossoming. Volunteers, interested researchers and experts from all corners of the globe were offering themselves to lead new review groups. By this time, more than 20 review groups were registered.

Many of those who attended the Oslo Colloquium have memories that hover around three distinct things: how expensive it was (one person remembers paying $30 for a bowl of soup); how isolating and unremitting the setting was (in a beautiful but cloud-enshrouded hotel on a mountain outside the city); and how a nasty – but possibly well-deserved – attack on the leadership of this young organization created a temporary crisis.

As mentioned earlier, the members of the Steering Group all had history with each other, and all were on a first-name basis. First names worked well in a small rebel army, especially one populated by people who had no use for ranks and hierarchies. In this fledgling organization, the main thing that distinguished you was your ability to follow through on what you had volunteered to do. Those who bit off large chunks and proved able to chew them earned admiration. Others, who liked the idea of hitching their wagon to this star, but weren't the completion types, filtered themselves out. Calling your friends Peter and Andy and Taddy (Kay Dickersin's nickname) and Brian and Dave was alright, and efficient. After all, it's better to use one word than two when you're in full sprint for an airplane taking off.

Jini Hetherington remembers Oslo well.[54] She said that the first two meetings of the new Collaboration (in Oxford and in Hamilton) were smaller affairs, but Oslo was a larger forum, with many newcomers curious to learn what this Cochrane thing was all about. She remembers the fog, the pricey drinks, and most of all, someone who stood up and confronted the Steering Group, saying, "Who are you and why do you keep referring to each other by your first names? Dave? Who's Dave?" This feeling escalated as others rose to question and challenge the Steering Group.

Hetherington explained: "Those people – Chris Silagy, Iain Chalmers, Brian Haynes – all referred to each other by first names. People who were newcomers, of course, felt excluded." It was pretty clear from the congregation of dissatisfied people that things got tense.

She wasn't the only one at that Oslo meeting who found herself shedding tears in the women's room, uncomfortable with the way things were turning ugly. There were others, too, frustrated both with the way the meeting was turning out and the way many of the female contributors felt marginalized.

Kay Dickersin remembers that there was also laughter coming from the women's room because, as they commiserated, they realized, in Kay's words, that even though the women might be accustomed to being excluded, "Now we were a big enough group that men were excluded from our tears and frustrations!"[55]

With the Steering Group in the main hall, sitting on the hot seat, Jini Hetherington recalled that the gathered mob was bluntly asserting the kinds of questions you'd get at the beginning of any new group, about governance and democracy. People were wondering who was leading this organization, who put them there, and the real question: "If we don't like you, how can we get rid of you?"

For Hetherington and others, this event signaled a major turning point in the history of the Cochrane Collaboration. She said, "After that Colloquium, the organization started to move to a more professional footing." One of the things that resulted from that meeting was the commitment to hold general elections every year, adopting what was seen as a formal democratic process to appointing the trustees.

Dave Sackett said that he was glad to be finishing his term as Chair of the Steering Group, though clearly it was still shaky and barely off the ground. He said, "It looked like the Collaboration would remain airborne, and now that its membership had burgeoned, it was time to begin to replace the volunteer launch party with elected members from the exciting, energetic gang who were clamoring to take over flying the enterprise." He said that it was good to be handing things over to others, so that it let him get back to his "primary Oxford job of trying to infect the UK and Europe with the EBM-bug," which he added, "wasn't a sure thing at that stage."

There is a certain nostalgia in looking back on the original group of insurgents. Hetherington told me, "Things were so exciting in those years, because if you wanted to do something, you could. You could make things happen. There was no bureaucracy. If you had a good idea, then the finger was pointed. Your idea. You do it. That was very rewarding."

The Oslo palace coup, while emotionally difficult for some, was fundamentally important. Dave Sackett admitted that it "represented a portion of the change from an appointed group to an elected group of leaders." The challengers from the floor also gave Sackett the chance to reiterate his thoughts to the crowd, the thought that everyone onboard was part of the crew of this airship. He told the assembly in Oslo that "You are far too preoccupied with people, and you are far too preoccupied with those of us who helped to get this thing going. We are not important. You are the important ones; not us. Cochrane is gonna succeed or fail on the basis of what you do. Not us."

Oslo was the meeting at which Sackett employed the notorious airplane analogy, which has since imprinted itself in the collective memory of the Cochrane Collaboration. He laughed, because he had used this analogy in other contexts.

He admitted that he might have used it when he was planning McMaster's medical curriculum in 1969 (after the first class had started the program). But in relation to the Oslo meeting, the airplane analogy suggested that this group was flying by the seat of its pants and that it was a work in progress. Basically, the plane was being built as it was taxiing down the runway. For him it was also part of signaling his handover, that it was "time for the passengers to take over, because its success or failure is gonna depend on what the passengers do. Not us."

At that meeting, Sackett officially completed his two years as Chair of the Steering Group and he stepped down as Chair. The Collaboration moved to an elected Steering Group – a natural development for a democratic, volunteer-based organization. His successor, the young, ambitious Chris Silagy, from Australia, was elected as Chair of the Steering Group.

Flying in Far-Flung Places

The year after the Cochrane Collaboration's launch, proof that the idea was "taking off" was manifest, with new centres being registered in Europe and in North America. Evidence-based health care was also gaining altitude in different forms. Interest in carrying out systematic reviews in all areas of medicine was spreading like a virus. One problem was that this Cochrane pandemic had yet to reach Australia or Asia. The most far-flung region and the most populous region on earth were, as yet, unrepresented in the Collaboration.

Maybe Chris Silagy was born to fix that deficit.[56] He was at least a generation younger than Dave Sackett, yet the one thing people said that he had in common with Sackett was his irreverence, which seemed to serve him well.

After the first Cochrane Colloquium, in 1993, Silagy had returned to Australia and gone to work, an evangelist for the cause of evidence-based medicine. He didn't seem to have much trouble getting Australians and New Zealanders enthused about this idea of the Collaboration.

Some have said that his youthful energy, equipped with lots of ideas, often caught people off-guard. People such as Caroline Crowther, his inaugural deputy director, and Sally Green, were with him right from the start and instrumental in developing the Australasian Cochrane Centre.[57]

Silagy was also crucial to the Collaboration's growth in other ways. As mentioned above, he became the first elected head of the Steering Group in its formative years (1996–98). He also travelled relentlessly, promoting the Collaboration worldwide and obtaining the funding it needed to move forward.

Iain Chalmers wrote that it was during Silagy's worldwide tour, drumming up interest in the Collaboration and establishing new networks, that Chris "first became troubled by symptoms of tiredness and lack of energy." What this turned out to be was the worst of all news: lymphoma.

Silagy's diagnosis of non-Hodgkin's lymphoma led to invasive treatments, including bone-marrow transplants and chemotherapy. Ironically, there was a dearth of information – comparative trials, for example – and large gaps in existing information. He wrote, "Sadly, even when I search the *Cochrane Library*, I find that the Collaboration is yet to establish a Haematological Malignancies Review Group."[58] It has one now, based in Cologne, Germany.

When Silagy handed over the Collaboration's reins in 1998, it was a much bigger and much healthier organization, one that Iain Chalmers said, "had a much clearer sense of identity and direction as a result of his efforts."

In March of 1998, Silagy delivered his Archie Cochrane Lecture at Green College, Oxford. The speech later became part of the introduction to the 1999 reprinting of Cochrane's book *Effectiveness and Efficiency*. In it, Silagy reveals the frustrations of being a patient. His most poignant message is that those who seek to provide good information to patients really need to listen to what those patients want. It's that simple.[59]

Silagy died in 2001 at age 41.

In honour of Chris Silagy, a prize is awarded every year at the Cochrane Colloquium to an individual who "has made an 'extraordinary' contribution to the work of the Cochrane Collaboration." It's usually a person who works behind the scenes; who makes things happen – someone who doesn't publish reviews; someone who is not a public figure for the Collaboration, but someone who, nevertheless, consistently contributes to the 'spirit of collaboration', the glue that holds the organization together.

Remaining Airborne

So, what helped the Cochrane Collaboration get airborne and stay that way? Sackett said that the evidence-based medicine movement and "this combination of key opinion leaders and senior clinicians, plus the fashion on which it was taken over by the young folks, certainly promoted its popularity and acceptance by clinicians."

Sackett claimed that his involvement with the Collaboration was a relic of ancient history, and that examining it now, from the perspective of his last Colloquium in Stavanger, Norway, in 2002, had little to do with the Collaboration of today. He made the point quite forcefully that "the important people in the Cochrane Collaboration are the folks out there, checking the journals, doing the analyses, trudging day-by-day; not folks like me."

Oslo happened over twenty years ago. That event is slipping into the mists of time. When I went to interview him in 2013, Sackett and his wife Barbara were nicely settled at Irish Lake in Canada, where he, despite official retirement from Oxford and from McMaster, continued to teach clinical trial methods, hold workshops, and help students and colleagues design and run randomized clinical trials. He wasn't active in the Collaboration, but he occasionally heard about how others were piloting the plane from his friends at the Canadian Cochrane Centre, now based in Ottawa.[60]

Sackett didn't attend a Colloquium since Stavanger. It was hard to prise him away from his cozy home at the edge of the lake. I asked him if he could be enticed to go to Quebec City for the twentieth anniversary celebrations in September, 2013. He abhorred going places where there was a risk he'd be recognized. He didn't need that. He joked that he'd only go to a future

Colloquium incognito, perhaps dressed in the gorilla suit he kept in his closet for formal occasions.

Sadly, he didn't get the chance: David Sackett died on May 13, 2015 in Markdale, Ontario.

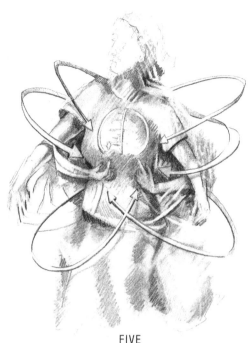

FIVE

The High Human Cost
of Not Acting on Quality Research

*"I would gladly have sacrificed my freedom
for a little knowledge."*

— Archie Cochrane,
*Effectiveness and Efficiency:
Random Reflections on Health Services*

IN THE SUMMER of 2012, the widest circulation newspaper in
the United States, *USA Today*[61] said that "75% of the world's 1
million preterm deaths could be avoided if a few 'proven and inexpensive' treatments and preventions" were widely available in
low-income countries. The article said that parents should learn

about "kangaroo care": mothers holding their babies in skin-to-skin contact for warmth in the absence of incubators. Also, it said that for women at risk of premature labor, a steroid injection costing about US $1 would help the immature lungs of their babies to develop, thus helping to prevent deaths and future respiratory problems.

It's not that the world doesn't have proven treatments. It's that we aren't adequately ensuring that people can get them.

Preterm birth kills approximately 1 million babies per year. It is the second leading cause of childhood death. The World Health Organization defines preterm as birth at or before 37 weeks of completed gestation. A full-term baby is usually born around 40 weeks, and according to the report *Born Too Soon: The Global Action Report on Preterm Birth,*[62] the risk of death for babies born at 37 to 39 weeks of gestation is twice as high as for full-term babies. That one or two weeks can make an enormous difference. Those premature babies who don't die shortly after birth are at risk of being disabled for life.

UN Secretary-General Ban Ki-moon wrote in the foreword to this report: "Let's change the future for millions of babies born too soon. The 'fundamental reality' is that this effort lacks the will, not the techniques, technologies or science. We know what to do. And we all have a role to play." [63] He made a good point about the technology and the science. The Cochrane Collaboration has played a key role in identifying these "proven treatments."

Of Sheep and Preterm Births

In 2001, the University of Auckland established a major research institute dedicated to fetal and child health. They named it the Liggins Institute after Sir Graham "Mont" Liggins, who was an obstetrician and researcher who wondered why babies often died when they had been born too soon.

Liggins wrote a letter to Iain Chalmers explaining how it was that he came to start researching the subject of preterm birth:[64]

When I returned to a position as Senior Lecturer in Obstetrics and Gynaecology at the National Women's Hospital in 1959, after six years of clinical work and no research in the UK, I realized that my academic appointment required me to do some research. I asked my friend, Bill Liley, of fetal transfusion fame, how to choose a topic. He said to look for a major problem which was potentially soluble. The major problem was easy. Prematurity stood out above everything else. I naively thought that all I had to do was solve the ancient question of what controlled the onset of labor at term and the reason for premature onset would become apparent.

What follows is an extraordinary story. It helped that Mont Liggins was a New Zealander, and that New Zealand has a lot of sheep, as well as a lot of sheepdogs. Sometimes, lambs are born too early because the mother ewes are stressed from being barked at and snapped at by the dogs.

The legend goes[65] that one of Liggins' neighbors, a sheep farmer, wondered why when dogs worry the ewes, their newborn lambs often die after premature delivery. Liggins reckoned it might have something to do with the steroid cortisol, released by a mammal under stress.

With a few experiments in sheep, he figured that labor is triggered by fetal cortisol release. He also noticed, in post mortem experimentation, that "the lungs of premature lambs normally sank in water because they had failed to fill with air. However, if the ewe had been given corticosteroids prior to delivery, the lungs inflated normally and would float. The steroids had stimulated production of a soapy substance, surfactant, vital for lung aeration."[66] Since this seemed to be the case for sheep, there was no reason to believe that it was not also for human newborns.

Liggins wanted to study the problem further. He enlisted a

neonatal colleague, Ross Howie, and they worked out a study design. They didn't know how much of the steroid to give mothers, but in his letter to Iain Chalmers, he indicates that they chose cortisone acetate. He wrote:

The choice of active agent came down to what drug company was willing to supply the active and placebo ampoules. Glaxo, originally a New Zealand company, came up trumps and the trial soon began. Glaxo could see that no profit was to be made, but were happy to do it for goodwill. It was by chance, then, that our choice of agent has turned out to be the best.[67]

The year was 1969, and they recruited 287 mothers in 22 months. The trial was a success. The survival rate of the newborns in the steroid group was much greater than that of the placebo group. Early neonatal mortality was 15 per cent in the control group, but only 3.2 per cent among the treated women.

He recalled, "We offered our manuscript first to *Nature*, which promptly rejected it without sending it out for review on the grounds that it lacked general interest." It was also rejected by *The Lancet*.[68] It was eventually published in 1972 in the journal *Pediatrics*.[69]

One researcher who found this study and became interested in steroid research for preterm infants was Dr. Patricia Crowley, a young Irish obstetrician. While this early steroid research was becoming known to the wider world, she had some real-world experience of premature infants. She'd seen a premature baby in her care die from respiratory distress.[70]

She explained that she was working at a London hospital, and her boss was starting a journal of obstetrics and gynaecology. She said, "The journal had received a paper disputing the value of antenatal steroids, and the editor asked me, 'Do you want to see if you could write a response to this paper?'" That inspired her to start looking in earnest for randomized trials of steroids, and it was about 1980 when, she said, she put them in "sort of a primitive table."

She continued. "I'd heard of Iain [Chalmers], and I went to visit him in Oxford in 1980 to see if I could have an attachment at the National Perinatal Epidemiology Unit [NPEU]. He was thinking of writing a book on effective care in labor and delivery." She said that he asked her to collaborate on that project.

Crowley was happy to work with Chalmers: "I was excited to have that attachment to NPEU in Oxford, and around about that time, the paper was published in the journal, and then we went to find more trials. I was going to write the chapter on antenatal steroids in the *ECPC* book."[71] Originally, it was going to be a small book, but eventually it grew into a large, two-volume tome.

Crowley: "So then I spent from September, 1980 to June, 1981 studying at the NPEU, and also doing a course in epidemiology in London and working on what became two chapters, on the induction of labor and on antenatal steroids. And about the same time, the collection of getting the trials together for the *Oxford Database of Perinatal Trials* was starting up. The trials I needed for these two chapters were being identified."

That was also when Mark Starr and his Update Software team were beginning to create computer-generated tables. Crowley recalls, "When the software was being tried out, the steroid trial was the first meta-analysis to be used in it."

Her review covered eight large trials, focusing on the use of steroids in prenatal care for women at risk of having preterm babies. As important as the evidence was in itself, the review has gone on to have a lasting Cochrane legacy: some of its results are depicted in the center of the Cochrane Collaboration's logo.

Iain Chalmers says of the logo:

Part of the [Cochrane] Centre's logo shows the results of the first seven trials of prenatal corticosteroids. I overlooked, inadvertently, an eighth trial that had been published during this time period. It happened to have exactly the same confidence interval as one of the others, and I had thought that we might have been double counting. The reason that we used the steroid trials was that we wanted to show that, within ten years of the Liggins and Howie trial, there had been crystal-clear evidence that this was a very important way of reducing neonatal deaths.

In launching the Cochrane Centre, we wanted to make the point that this very important information had been available more than a decade earlier. Yet, it was still not being acted upon sufficiently in practice.

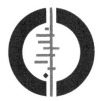

Soon the logo of the Cochrane Centre was appearing in brochures and presentations. It was particularly useful in describing the objectives of the Cochrane Centre in the UK and, later, the international Cochrane Collaboration.

In Chalmers' words, through this one review, "We made the point that tens of thousands of babies had suffered and died unnecessarily (and cost health services more than they need have done) because information had not been assembled in a systematic review and meta-analysis to show the strength of the evidence."

When you think of Liggins and Howie's research in 1972, then of Patricia Crowley's somewhat primitive systematic review in the early 1980s, and then of the definitive logo-centered systematic review that emerged from Mark Starr's software in 1991, it's clear that a lot of time elapsed. In fact, between the earliest study and a high-quality systematic review of the use of antenatal corticosteroid therapy, nearly 20 years had passed. And it wasn't until 1994 that the US National Institutes of Health produced a consensus statement recommending the use of corticosteroids for preterm infants. That's more than two decades after Liggins and Howie's work.

It wouldn't surprise Roger Soll that it took a while for this new research to be put into practice. He knew all about newborn babies, a field known as neonatology. Soll is a professor at the University of Vermont, a pediatrician in the Department of Pediatrics, and he's been with the Cochrane Collaboration since its inception. He's been doing neonatal research since before the Collaboration started.[72]

Soll's group focuses on the health of newborns, a field called neonatology, and he thought that if Iain Chalmers could do what he did with obstetrics, then it was a "natural thing to extend to the neonate after that."

Soll: "I met [Chalmers] back then, with his huge file cabinet of cards, pre-computer, and he was a huge influence on me." Also influential in Soll's life were Jack Sinclair and Mike Bracken, whose book *Effective Care of the Newborn Infant*[73] was a "direct follow-on from the big two-volume set produced by Murray Enkin, Marc Keirse and Iain Chalmers."

Soll reminded me that giving birth to a baby before its time can be deadly. He said, "Somewhere around one in ten babies are delivered what they call 'preterm', and that's not good. Many of those babies will suffer from a condition called respiratory distress syndrome (RDS) and many will either die or be seriously harmed by it. RDS can affect nearly half the babies born before 30 weeks."

He knew of Liggins and Howie's work and is able to give it some context: "Since the early 1970s, it was known from animal experiments, and even the first human trial, that if you gave corti-costeroid medications to mothers who threatened to deliver pre-term, that it absolutely reduced the incidence of breathing problems in the newborn, and even death. These studies were done in the 1970s. Study after study was done in the '70s and in the '80s."

Medical Caprice, Infant Mortality

But did those studies change what physicians did? Not right away. When it comes to evidence, why do some people ignore it and others only take what they want?

Then there are questions about the quality of the individual studies. Soll said, "Of course, some studies were not powered to have the appropriate sample size. Some did not quite show a statistically significant result, and the interpretation in the obstetric field was more like a Rorschach test. People looked at [these] data and they did whatever they wanted to do [according to] whatever they saw in it."

In the real world, that meant that some mothers at risk of having a pre-term baby did not get the treatment. Babies who didn't have to die were dying. It's one thing to have an effective drug that works. It's another thing to ignore the evidence that proves that the drug works. Why does this happen: that we have a drug that works but isn't used?

Soll explained: "The big complaint is that people 'cherry pick' the evidence. They don't look at it all; they don't look at it in context. [However], in fact, there are rather simple and straight-forward statistical techniques that allow you to synthesize it and get a much more precise answer."

"Sometimes," he continued, "people choose the study which they're familiar with. Maybe it's from a major journal. Maybe it's from their country. Maybe it's in their language. There's also a fear of change. I mean, we all have a great deal of our own personal psychology involved in this."

He told me one of the problems at that time: that giving drugs to pregnant women had a particularly bad taint to it, owing to the recent experience with thalidomide (which caused disfiguring birth defects) and DES (diethylstilbestrol) which was thought at the time to prevent miscarriages, but which caused unusual reproductive tract cancers in the children, particularly the female children of the mothers who took it. This problem was only identified decades later, and so caution about giving any treatment during pregnancy was probably heightened.

Soll laments the high human cost of not acting on quality research as it begins to accumulate: "And so, in fact, less than one in five preterm infants, even… ten years after this first trial, was being born after their mothers had been treated with ante natal steroids… one out of five possible candidates for this lifesaving drug."

A Challenge to Change

Some people observing Iain Chalmers at the time said that he wasn't hesitant to speak or write about what Cochrane's logo meant, and that he wasn't afraid to speak forcefully.[74] It was as if the logo was a big hammer, and perhaps everything looked like a nail.

As Soll said, "He didn't just present the data scientifically and say, 'Well, let the community do what it may.' He really spoke to the fact that this evidence needs to be acted on." Soll explained that Chalmers told his audiences, "'We need to react to it. What are you gonna do about it?' He used [the logo] to disseminate the idea of meta-analysis and he challenged people."

Soll saw Chalmers out there issuing this challenge: "Are you gonna practise evidence-based medicine? Here's a perfect example of it! Are you going to change?"

Change started to occur, but it was slow. Soll said it really helped when "eventually major national organizations got behind [steroid use], and made workshops with guideline statements [based] on it." The results have been fabulous. "We've gone from a 15 per cent to 20 per cent usage to well into the 80 per cent usage. So [steroid use has] quadrupled since that work."

Read My _____

The Cochrane logo has been seen everywhere: on mugs, on posters, in presentations, and on T-shirts. Possibly its most memorable use occurred in 1996 at the Colloquium in Adelaide, Australia.

The logo appeared on a T-shirt worn by Patricia Crowley as she debated the value of evidence-based health care. Back then, the concept might have been new enough to be subject to debate, but this particular debate was intended to provide lighthearted amusement for the delegates. The title of the debate: "Within ten years, all healthcare decisions will be evidence-based."

There were three speakers for the motion, and three against it. The moderator was Jini Hetherington, who wore a black gown and was there to keep the peace. Unlike the year before, in Oslo, the mood in Adelaide was upbeat and fun. This was the final event of the Colloquium, and was meant to leave the delegates informed, amused and energized. Crowley said, "We had the easy side, as it was easy to show how observational evidence was shown to be biased."

Few people remember the substance of the debate, but they do remember Crowley's punchline. As her closing point, to make her case for the importance of systematic reviews in advancing human health, she pointed to the Cochrane logo on her T-shirt and most infamously said, "If you don't believe what I've been saying, read my tits."

And, like the logo, you don't soon forget the effect of those words.

Benefits and Harms

There is another subchapter to the corticosteroids story. It reminds us that any technology we use must be continually monitored to make sure that the benefits outweigh the harms.

Roger Soll says, "OK, you've got a premature baby. The story is corticosteroids again. For Iain, it was before birth, and for us it was after birth. In much higher doses, corticosteroids came into use to decrease lung inflammation."

Soll continued: "If you put babies on a breathing machine, it damages their lungs. It sets up a cycle of inflammation that causes a good deal of this lung damage. In the first trials of corticosteroids in babies at risk of developing this lung damage that we call bronchopulmonary dysplasia, steroids were incredibly effective. They decreased the need for supplemental oxygen; they tended towards decreasing death; they were hugely effective." That was, he said, "until we pieced it together in the review and we started to look at some of the harms that were further downstream. So it turns out that, in the studies that were coming out, and as we pieced it together in – through – the reviews, they had a much higher rate of cerebral palsy."

He points out that, when the early trials were coming out, post-natal steroid use "was about 30 percent in very low birth [weight] infants."

And then, after the early follow-up trials and a review in the *Cochrane Library*, Soll said, "It was very clear. There was a much-increased risk of cerebral palsy." Later, he said, "The Academy of Pediatrics, the Canadian Pediatric Society, all came out with strong statements about how this drug should be used sparingly, if at all. It's dropped down to 8 per cent. That was somewhere around the late 1990s, I believe."

Seek the Rationale

If you are reading this, it's because you're alive. And you might be alive because your mother did something really important to you as a baby. She put you down to sleep on your back. Now that might seem trivial, but sometimes it's the smallest of things that make the biggest of differences.

I slept on my back as a baby. I know, because I once asked my mother about this. She said that when we (my brother and two sisters) were babies she always put us on our backs in the crib. To her, that was normal: "It just seemed the right thing to do."

"But what about Dr. Spock?" I asked.

I was being a little devious. I was asking my mom a loaded question.

I was referring to Dr. Benjamin McLane Spock, the American pediatrician and author of probably the most influential baby care book ever written. In fact his *Common Sense Book of Baby and Child Care*[75] (first published in 1946) was considered in its time to be the absolute bible on babies. It sold more copies than any other book in the world in the latter half of the 20th century. Only the real Bible sold more copies. Everyone having babies after the war would have heard of Dr. Spock, even my mother, who like many women at the tail end of the post-war baby boom were hungry for expert baby advice as they went forth to multiply.

Back in 1963 asnooze in a crib (on my back), little did I know that my mother was being a renegade – because the respected Dr. Spock told parents to put babies to sleep on their fronts.

"I didn't like that advice, so I ignored it," my mom explains matter-of-factly.

But Dr. Spock was *an expert*. In fact he was *the* expert of my mom's generation. His argument seemed solid enough: If babies vomit, as babies frequently do, they would choke on their vomit and stop breathing. Many would die. Who was to argue with him? Crib death, or cot death as it was called, is a common cause of death for infants. There are many theories to try to explain why babies sometimes unexpectedly die in the crib, but Dr.

Spock's front-sleeping expert advice was delivered to millions of parents around the world. Many people would heed this advice.

Problem was, even the world's biggest baby authority, the expert's expert, the guy who wrote the bible on baby care was wrong. Dead wrong. Numerous meta-analyses since that time have proven that sleeping on their backs was safer for babies.[76]

The lesson here is not: "Don't listen to experts".

The lesson here is: "Don't listen to experts who have no evidence." In other words, expert advice is unreliable if it comes unattached to any research, or any proof, that the advice is reliable. If the advice is coming from the land of uncertainty, that needs to be made clear. If there is some research that supports the expert's opinion, is it reliable, high quality and useful? If not, maybe more and better research is required.

What is clear is that before recommending any kind of 'treatment' there should be some assurance that the benefits exceed the harms.

Dr. Benjamin Spock's famous key message to mothers was: "Trust yourself. You know more than you think you do." I take some solace from the fact that my mother seemed to know enough to avoid one bit of advice from an 'expert' physician.

Not all healthcare decisions are a question of life and death. As Cochrane has been able to demonstrate, many of the things that can help us have good evidence behind them.

But there is also a tendency to pick the facts we like; to follow our gut instincts, which is what my mother did. Following our instincts or following the experts may lead us in the wrong direction. This is why I believe if the world didn't have an entity to collect, sift and assess evidence, we'd have to invent one. Once you understand what evidence can do, you may never lie down in your bed the same way again.

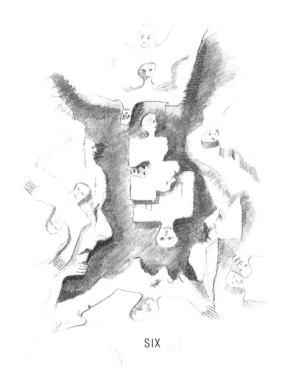

SIX

Connecting with Consumers

"Right at the very beginning, when the idea was getting peddled, a lot of people said, 'This is too high risk. Don't get involved with this madcap scheme.' And some people even said to me, 'You'll ruin your reputation, Hilda! Don't do it!'"

— Hilda Bastian, Cochrane's first consumer advocate

WHEN MARYANN NAPOLI attended her first Cochrane Colloquium in Lyons, France, in October, 2001, she was in for some surprises. Napoli had co-founded the Center for Medical Consumers in New York City in 1976, and had been familiar with the work of the Collaboration for several years. Even so, she remembers that Cochrane was still capable of the unexpected.[77]

Cochrane's annual Colloquium takes place in a different city every September/October. It can be intense. The days often start off with breakfast meetings at 7 AM and continue with workshops and plenary sessions, with a few more meetings crammed in at the end. It's not unusual to spend 12 hours a day in meetings at a Cochrane Colloquium, and there is a strong draw to be out mixing in the crowds, finally putting a face to the name of someone, for example, whom you've worked with only by e-mail for two years. The evenings might have parties and more meetings – a schedule that can exhaust even the fittest.

When Maryann Napoli was in Lyons, she happened into a particular workshop where she was astounded to learn something she'd never heard before: that when drug trials are concluded, the harms data – that is, the information about who was hurt, how they were hurt, and perhaps how many died – are often either not recorded or not included in the published results.

She said, "I had been a medical writer reporting to the lay public for over 20 years, by then. Yet this was entirely new to me. When I returned to New York, I told every seasoned consumer advocate I knew, including people who had served on FDA drug advisory panels. No one had ever heard it before!"

To her, this was all the more shocking because the US drug marketing machine seemed no longer to focus primarily on sick or even elderly people. "From the pharmaceutical industry's point of view, the ideal drug customers are healthy adults in early middle age, willing to go on long-term drug therapy for risk factors like high cholesterol, low bone density and pre-hypertension," said Napoli. Those otherwise healthy people were her constituency.

A Work in Progress

Napoli is not your average consumer advocate. Nor is she your average Cochrane consumer[78]. Unlike most consumers who arrive at the Collaboration because of a deep interest in a specific disease and an interest in volunteering to make a difference, Napoli's concern is healthy individuals turned into patients before their time. As she told me, with a hint of irony, "You'd better be more careful about any medical intervention when you're healthy, symptom free, and kept in the dark about harms, because you've got more to lose."

Napoli strives to make sure that consumers understand the pros and cons of treatment. She was at the forefront in calling public attention to the risks of mammography screening in the 1970s, when it was introduced to American women. She had initially heard of the Cochrane Collaboration because she found herself carrying on a one-woman promotion of evidence-based medical care to the public. But back then, she said, "You really didn't use the word 'evidence.'"

She accepts that the word *evidence* might now carry a negative connotation or be misleading, but for her it's a simple proposition: Does the information given to me by my doctor about treatments include proof that it is effective? In her words, "Does this work? And for whom is it proven to be effective?"

Napoli likes to experiment with her friends to see to what degree they are being sucked in, confused, or biased by medical advice. She generally finds enough to disturb. Her friends, she says, are smart and worldly, and able to see through the public relations spin and promotional bumph surrounding many things, but she often finds that the messages emerging from good quality research are not getting through.

For example, she'll ask her friends simple questions: "Do you take statins [cholesterol-lowering drugs]? Why? What do you expect from them?" Simple questions, but the answers often confuse her.

"They'll say, '[They're] very good for lowering my cholesterol,'" she says. "And I'll come back and say, 'But what's the reason you're taking [them]? Not just to lower your cholesterol.' And they are stumped."

The real reason, perhaps obvious to Napoli, that anyone takes statins is to decrease their chances of having a heart attack or a stroke. That's what the drugs are supposed to do. But instead, she says, most people focus on their cholesterol levels.

This tendency is what's known as a surrogate endpoint, which might have nothing to do with a drug's main purpose. She says, "That's the point of view brought to you by the drug industry, especially when you're in a country like ours where they are advertising to you directly. And they are training us. And that's what disappoints me."

Napoli had heard about the work of Iain Chalmers and his colleagues before this organization called the Cochrane Collaboration existed – some time in the 1980s, when she was looking at interventions used in pregnancy and childbirth. She read a review of all the interventions – "everything from the dipstick in the urine when you're first pregnant to things like fetal monitoring" – and was stunned to learn that the 500-or-so interventions lined up this way: "A third of them had really good data to support that they worked; that the benefits outweighed the risks. There was another third... in the gray area, and we didn't know one way or another. The last third [were] outright dangerous, and they were still doing [them]."

As a medical writer, Napoli depends on others to produce reliable information. It was the independent, solid analyses of the research behind medical interventions that drew her to the Collaboration, but it took a while before she became anything more than a user of Cochrane reviews.

She drew inspiration and encouragement from Cochrane leaders such as Peter Gøtzsche in Copenhagen (Nordic Cochrane Centre), Tom Jefferson in Rome (vaccines field), and Jim Wright in Vancouver (Hypertension Review Group). All were in the forefront of acknowledging the problems of the industry-funded trials that formed the basis of their respective Cochrane reviews. All were vocal about missing harms data. Napoli wanted to see these issues addressed, where relevant, in what is often the only part of a Cochrane review read by consumers: the brief précis at the beginning, known as the plain language summary (PLS).

After the Lyons Colloquium, Napoli's advocacy within the Collaboration soon focused on improving the PLSs. These are aimed at the general public and omit a lot of information. In her opinion, they aren't as good as they need to be. "Why," she wondered, "are most PLSs so deficient, especially in addressing the harms of drugs and other medical interventions? Why do Cochrane drug reviews fail to disclose industry sponsorship of the [included] trials? Why don't they state the size of the drug's benefit?"

Napoli took years to understand how the Collaboration works and to learn the steps needed to persuade such a large organization to make major changes in the abstracts and PLSs of its reviews. With the help of others in the Cochrane Consumer Network, most notably Janet Wale and Silvana Simi, she began to explore ways to make improvements. She decided that, in the Cochrane way, she needed to collect some evidence to support their case.

For example, how about doing a survey to find out if Cochrane drug reviews mentioned industry sponsorship of the included trials? "The idea for this survey came to me around 2004, when I noticed a rare mention of commercial sponsorship of included trials... in a Cochrane review about breakfast cereals." That led to a Colloquium poster, coauthored with Janet Wale, about the widespread failure to disclose industry sponsorship of the trials included in Cochrane drug reviews.

As part of her mission to make changes, Napoli went the Colloquium route with workshops, more posters, and even tried (unsuccessfully) to get the issue on the Steering Group meeting agenda in 2007. With encouragement from the US Cochrane Center, she sent an open letter to *Cochrane Library* Editor in Chief David Tovey, signed by other consumers, calling for specific improvements to the abstracts and the PLSs. By July 2011, the time had come for the Collaboration to address these issues.

The letter happened to coincide with the US National Library of Medicine's offer to include Cochrane PLSs along with abstracts online at PubMed Health, a new consumer-oriented tool for locating evidence-based medicine. As a result, the abstracts and PLSs began to receive the attention they deserved. Pretty important, especially given that many people, including practicing physicians, read no further.

Napoli now serves on a Cochrane committee that started work in January, 2012 to revise PLS standards. The committee's work continues.

Everyone, it seems, agrees that the PLS is a work in progress, including David Tovey, the Collaboration's first-ever editor in chief.

Based in London, Tovey joined the Collaboration in 2009. He has demonstrated a keen interest in making sure that Cochrane reviews meet high standards, as well as serving all the necessary constituencies: policymakers, clinicians *and* consumers.[79]

Tovey is involved in increasing the relevance of the PLS. He told me, "The Cochrane [review authors] historically tend to concentrate on the methods of conducting the review," so this involves lots of detail and quantitative language. However, he says, "The [PLSs] and abstracts are the parts of Cochrane reviews that will be by far the most read and, to some extent, they can be seen as the icing on the cake." There certainly is a balancing act, as the whole review really contains the substance of the research. If you only look at the PLS, you might be missing out.

He added, "I think, to be fair, we need to increase the quality and consistency of [PLS], and we also need to think about whether there are communication methods that we're not employing that could improve them further."

Making Medicine "Very Patient Centered"

Many of the consumers who join the Collaboration as contributors feel driven to it by an illness of their own, belong to a health charity that supports people with a particular illness (such as arthritis), or are caregivers who want to bring the patient's and caregiver's perspective to the Collaboration's work.

Silvana Simi came to the Collaboration through a different route than Napoli. Simi, who lives in Italy, has a daughter with multiple sclerosis (MS), a debilitating nervous system disease.[80]

She explains: "One day, by chance, I was looking on the internet, and I saw this Cochrane Multiple Sclerosis [Review] Group. I [had] never heard about the Cochrane [Collaboration]. I thought I was a well-informed researcher, but apparently I was not." Fortunately for her, Simi found that the MS Review Group had its editorial base in Italy, so she called Milan. That's how her involvement began.

For Simi, joining the Collaboration was "simply a way to fight my private war against MS." She went on later to serve for three years as a consumer representative on the Collaboration's Steering Group. Her commitment is straightforward: "I want to make medicine very patient centered." She wants to ensure that good quality information gets to patients, and that people with diseases "speak up for themselves." What this means in practise is that she spends a lot of time in the MS community, learning what MS patients want and need. A central question she often asks is,

"Are their preferences reflected in the research being done, and if not, how can we change that?"

Being both a researcher and a patient advocate has given Simi the unusual ability to consider both researchers' and patients' needs simultaneously. She has gone beyond the MS community, and her role as patient advocate extends to all areas of consumer health care.

One of her roles is to act as a "consumer referee" for systematic reviews. Does a review make sense? Is it meaningful to consumers? If it isn't helpful, how can it be made so? Simi is also aware of the problems of living in a non-English-speaking country and works to help translate the plain language summaries into Italian.

Australian consumer advocate Janet Wale is a hardcore consumer participant in the Collaboration. She has worked alongside people like Napoli and Simi for over a decade.

Wale is most closely associated with the Cochrane Consumer Network (CCNet), created in 1996 to formalize the involvement of consumers in the Collaboration. She was part of an initiative to find out what the authors of Cochrane reviews wanted from consumers.

The findings from that survey, carried out by external consultants and published in 2009, provided some needed support for consumer involvement. It concludes that review authors want consumers to help improve the readability and quality of reviews, and to improve the usefulness of the PLSs. This was perhaps a perennial recognition that the scientists and review authors who put together reviews need the different skill set (and perspective) that only consumers can provide.

Risky Business, Leaky Pipes

What keeps consumers interested in the Collaboration? Napoli says that one thing she admires about the Collaboration is the willingness of its people to confront problems head on. She says,

"There are all these wonderful people coming together who are blowing the whistle, essentially, on the quality of trials, and they are trying to improve them as they go on." In her mind, however, she focuses on the main thing that matters to her: how will all this ultimately help consumers?

One "distortion" that frustrates her is the way statistics are used to mislead people. She points to how relative versus absolute differences in a drug's effects are conveyed. By way of example, she talks about a drug called alendronate, or Fosamax, an osteoporosis drug that has been a leader for many years in a class of drugs called bisphosphonates.

Napoli explained that when the first drug in that class came on the market, about 20 years ago, it was approved on the basis of a trial in elderly women considered at "high risk" for fractures. Participants were randomly assigned to a placebo or Fosamax. The authors reported that, after 3 years, there was a "50% reduction in risk of hip fracture" for women taking the drug compared to placebo. Napoli said somewhat mockingly, "Didn't that sound fabulous?" Her eyes narrowed as she went on. "And wouldn't you be suicidal not to take this drug because that sounds really good?" But there's more to the story.

"So here's what [that] means in absolute terms," she said. "In the women who were randomly assigned to Fosamax, only 1 percent of that group had a hip fracture at three years, compared to 2 percent of the women who did nothing. I don't think that the public really understands how minimal that is, and one reason they don't is because I, as a consumer advocate, would turn that stat[istic] around and say, 'Look at this: 98 percent of these high-risk elderly women did *not* have a hip fracture in the next three years.'"

That's not the message coming out, especially to those people exposed to the ubiquitous drug advertisements in magazines and on TV in the USA. The reality, she explains, is that maybe 1 per cent of women who take this drug for three years will be prevented from having a hip fracture. Since 1 per cent is half of 2 per cent ("50% less" than 2 per cent), guess what stat gets used in the advertisements, in the medical journal articles and, unfortunately, in Cochrane abstracts? Yes! This drug will reduce hip fractures by 50 per cent! Understanding drug effects is all about understanding percentages.

Does the drug help 1 per cent of people or 50 per cent? Napoli says, "I cannot understand why the Collaboration hangs on to the use of relative risks in their use of abstracts when we know that the public, as well as clinicians, misinterpret that." We also know that these "relative risk reductions" are often presented in statistics that exaggerate the effects of a treatment, leaving both physicians and patients with the impression that a drug is much more effective than it actually is.

Napoli and her consumer advocate colleagues don't want the Collaboration to report these large and misleading relative risk reductions. But with this issue, as with many others, changing the methods of a large organization – even the Cochrane Collaboration – doesn't happen overnight.

She said, "First I had to explain it; kind of convince fellow advocates… and then you have to convince the Collaboration to change the [*Cochrane Handbook for Systematic Reviews of Interventions*]."[81] She went on, "A lot of us don't understand relative risk, and when you use that, you are basically giving information that serves the drug industry's interests, because they know as well as we do that we are overestimating the benefits when [they're] given in relative risk terms."

The Collaboration can count itself lucky that it has the help of seasoned consumer advocates like Maryann Napoli and Silvana Simi, who have been fighting for better PLSs, disclosure of drug industry funding of studies, and meaningful descriptions of drug effects. They have pushed the organization from within, and the

Collaboration does respond. Policies change, though sometimes slowly.

The battles fought by consumers within the Cochrane Collaboration might be emblematic of many fights within the research world, and within big organizations where the effort to make even the smallest of changes seem Herculean.

Everywhere in this organization, there are consumer advocates who see a major hole in the Collaboration's piping, and water gushing everywhere. When they start to fix it, they realize how hard it is to get people concerned about all the water pouring in, and to convince all the plumbers and pipefitters that they need to get to work. But they persist and work until the hole is plugged. And maybe, just as they're ready to rest, another pipe springs a leak, and the process begins anew. Luckily, the consumers within the Collaboration generally do find a welcome and receptive audience – people committed to working alongside consumers to get those leaks fixed.

Singing the Evidence

Godwin Aja is professor of Public Health at Babcock University in Nigeria.[82] He has seen other kinds of leaks that need fixing. He wants to find the best strategies for improving healthcare delivery in some of the poorest countries in the world, and spends a lot of time pushing against governments. It's what many consumer activists see as their key job: being a squeaky wheel that demands attention on the important matter of delivering health care.

Aja has been a member of the Cochrane Collaboration Steering Group, as well as a member of the CCNet executive committee, and says that, both in the developed and the developing world, "consumer issues are still not well addressed." He says, "There seems to be no clear interaction between government and consumer groups." It's a situation that mustn't continue, and something he desperately wants to change.

Aja first heard of the Cochrane Collaboration in 1998, as a member of Health Action International (HAI), an organization that promotes access to essential drugs and the provision of quality drug information. Through HAI, he was invited to his first Cochrane Colloquium in Rome in 1999. Hilda Bastian was working to recruit African consumers to join the Collaboration, and he thinks Bastian discovered that he was involved in HAI. As he explained, "She sent the Cochrane Consumer Network registration form to me to join. I am glad I did!"

Whether you are from Norway, New Hampshire or Nigeria, consumers face similar challenges – as Aja learned when he showed up in Rome. That Colloquium was an exciting and captivating experience for him – especially meeting consumers from around the globe and realizing that they had a lot in common.

He wants to involve more consumers in the Collaboration, to "bring consumer groups together and [persuade] them to raise the specific issues that affect them." He wants people in the villages and cities of Africa to be users, and perhaps creators, of evidence-based healthcare information.

One condition that affects many of the people living on that large, sprawling continent is malaria, a mosquito-borne disease and one of the world's biggest causes of premature death. Preventing malaria, which affects as many as 500 million people per year and causes as many as 2.7 million deaths (mostly of children), is a major public health challenge. As many as one in five childhood deaths in sub-Saharan Africa are attributed to malaria.[83] Fortunately, with cheap and readily available prevention in the form of bed nets, especially if the nets are treated with insecticide, many of those deaths could be prevented.

According to Aja, the evidence is clear "that insecticide-treated bed nets are a very useful intervention in malaria control," but there starts his challenge: How do you get that information, as well as the nets, out to local communities so they will start using them and saving lives?

He says, "A good number of Cochrane reviews exist that talk about the benefits of insecticide-treated bed nets." The question is one of translation: taking scientific information of high quality and making it accessible to the people who need it.

Many of the consumers in the Collaboration find their niche in doing translation: not just translating the scientific concepts into plain language, but putting the information into local languages, and even using more traditional and home-grown ways of communicating it.

In some countries, the concept of consumers is different from in the West. Professor Mingming Zhang is currently a consumer representative on the Steering Group who works in the West China Hospital in Sichuan University. She has been employed there since 1997 to help establish the Chinese Cochrane Centre.[84]

She said that, for the first six or seven years, "Our work was just dissemination, to raise awareness of what the Cochrane Collaboration means." But it wasn't dissemination to consumers; it was to health professionals in China who weren't aware of it and needed to have the benefits of systematic research explained. For her, this meant translating many of the more important Cochrane review abstracts into Chinese.

Over the years, Zhang has seen the effect of Cochrane reviews grow in China, but she wonders, "as a consumer advocate... how many reviews or how much Cochrane evidence really impacts clinical practice and improves patient outcomes?" For her, what's important is not the number of reviews used, but whether the reviews actually have influence.

She said that she wants to see Cochrane reviews form the basis of national guidelines in China – work that would really influence or guide physicians' behavior. She wants Cochrane reviews to be more widely known, and says, "As a non-English-speaking representative, I really hope to see some realistic strategies to improve the wider participation in the Collaboration of non-English speaking countries."

EVEN THOUGH access to *The Cochrane Library* is free in all developing countries, its contents are still out of reach to those who can't easily access computers or the internet. And then there is the appropriateness or helpfulness of the information. Godwin Aja reminded me that, even though he translates many PLS into local languages and shares them with consumer groups, they still might be hard to understand.

Aja said, "We operate in a culture where oral tradition is important, and people have their own way of learning." He has to use whatever means necessary, including storytelling, poems, even drama to convey the evidence. Aja has a method.

Armed with Cochrane evidence demonstrating the importance of insecticide-treated bed nets, he goes to rural villages and asks the local people for their help in animating it. He says, "We get them to use the evidence to generate the poems and the songs, with a drummer providing the beat." He has seen it work very well. He said, "At the end of the day, they own the evidence. They use it. They sing about it."

Singing about evidence? One might say that's a novel approach – but if it works, why not? Perhaps song is the ultimate medium for a Cochrane review. Involving consumers is more than just giving them information; it is attracting them to an alliance in which they understand the evidence and its lifesaving messages well enough to make them their own.

Home Birth or Hospital Birth?

One of the most important decisions a couple has to make when a baby is on the way is where the baby should be born. In a hospital? At home with a midwife? Or in some other kind of supportive environment? Where is it safest to deliver one's baby, and where can one find quality information to help make that decision?

If information is power, then sometimes the information available in Cochrane reviews can provide consumers with the power boost they need to combat irrational and occasionally inhuman healthcare practices.

Cochrane consumer advocate Alina Bishop Velarde has felt that power and she is using it to revolutionize how women give birth in Mexico. Velarde lives in Tepoztlán, Morelos, in central Mexico. She is a midwife and consumer advocate on the front lines in the battle to make childbirth safer for all women and their babies. She's been a member of the CCNet for over a decade and her group Parto Libre (PartoLibreMexico.org) works on educating women and lobbying governments. She says that among her biggest and best tools are systematic reviews produced by the Cochrane Collaboration.[85]

She explains, "Although pregnancy and childbirth health care is completely free in Mexico, public hospitals in Mexico are overloaded and lack sufficient resources. This leads to poor quality health care, partly because care during childbirth is not evidence-based, and hospitals still adhere to many practices not recommended by the World Health Organization."

Velarde tells me she had an "Oh my God" moment when she was invited to read and comment on a Cochrane review about traditional labor. The review was important for her because she was a traditional birth attendant trainer, and it reflected a problem that women in countries all around the world face: having adequately trained attendants help with their births.

For someone who is fighting for the rights of women to deliver their babies in non-medicalized, more traditional settings, any kind of scientific support would help. A Cochrane review, originally published in 1998 and updated in 2012, declared that "there is no strong evidence from randomized trials to favour either planned hospital birth or planned home birth for low-risk pregnant women."[86] It also says, "Increasingly, better observational studies suggest that planned hospital birth is not any safer than planned home birth assisted by an experienced midwife with collaborative medical back-up, but may lead to more interventions and more complications."

She told me that better access to midwives and better midwifery training are both important, but there are other factors – particularly related to poverty – that continue to have major effects on maternal mortality. This is perhaps reflected in the fact that almost 1,000 women per day around the world die from complications of pregnancy or childbirth.[87] Every year, more than a million children are left motherless due to death during or right after childbirth. Reducing the level of maternal mortality (mothers dying in childbirth) is one of the millennium development goals set by the World Health Organization (WHO).

Velarde's group, founded in Mexico in 2007, aims to make minimally-interventionist births more possible in that country. This fight is partly about giving midwives the respect she thinks they deserve, but it's a tough slog, especially facing a patriarchal and hierarchical medical system that pushes women into hospital deliveries because they are told that they are "safest." The answer for her: Find good quality evidence and use it to lobby for change.

When I met her in Madrid at the 2011 Cochrane Colloquium, Velarde told me about being asked to act as a consumer representative in discussions regarding the Reproductive Health Library (RHL) at the WHO. She was pleased to be one of four women (the others were from India, Africa and Australia) invited to review the RHL to see if it was serving the needs of the people on the receiving end of health care.

Essentially, the RHL is a repackaging of Cochrane reviews. It takes the best available evidence on sexual and reproductive health from Cochrane reviews and makes action-oriented suggestions both to clinicians (doctors and nurses) and to policymakers. It was new to her. "It was the first time I heard about a library being based on the reviews of the Cochrane [Collaboration]" and it was vitally important to her as a prenatal educator. In fact, she said that the Cochrane reviews gave her some ammunition she needed: to support and reinforce women's right to choose the kind of birth they want.

Through her work on the RHL, she became familiar with the Better Births Initiative in South Africa, which aims to help health professionals to access, understand, and use the information in the RHL. She found that the program wasn't available in Spanish, so she translated the materials, which focused on about a dozen Cochrane reviews which were aimed at improving care during childbirth. This has been a real catalyst for her in helping to "open doors to public health services in Mexico, and hospitals with training doctors and nurses."

For Velarde, having access to Cochrane reviews has also been vital in her discussions with Mexican government officials. She said, "We have specific contacts, friends in the medical field who are very hard at work on transforming the experience of childbirth for women."

Being part of the Cochrane Consumer Network, and working with consumer activists in other countries, such as Gill Gyte, Sonja Henderson and Tina Lavender, has been a real boon for Alina. When people from other countries come to your own country and demonstrate to your own officials the value of what you're doing, it helps immensely. She said that because Tina Lavender (one of the Pregnancy and Childbirth Group's editors) could attend a variety of international conferences (including one at the National Institute of Perinatology in Mexico), she had been able to highlight the importance of Velarde's work.

Sometimes, it's not just the work, but the network, that makes all the difference.

Evidence at Hand Changes Everything

Hilda Bastian has many claims to fame. She can say that she is one of the founders of the Cochrane Collaboration; at the first Colloquium, she was the only one from the southern hemisphere (she's Australian); she claims to have had less formal education than anyone else among the founding group (she's a high school dropout); and she was the first and, at that time, the only consumer advocate on the original Steering Group. She's a starter – a person who sees a need and makes things happen. Both the Plain Language Summaries (PLSs) and the Cochrane Consumer Network (CCNet) were among her initiatives. To round out her chops, she's also done her time as a coordinating editor of a Cochrane review group, and she was the editor of the international newsletter during the formative years.

You get a sense of the expansive kind of thinker Bastian is when she says, "The principles of evidence apply to everything." When it comes to health care, for her, "It's simple. It's about learning about what works."

Perhaps unaware that she sounds as though she's channeling the ghost of Archie Cochrane, she outlines her basic principles: "Learn from your mistakes and the mistakes of others. Learn from what works. Do something because it works, not just because it feels like the right thing to do because it's in your interests." And what is most important (and perhaps most Archie-esque) is this particular assertion: "Always think about the adverse effects – how things might go wrong."

Bastian was already doing extensive health consumer advocacy work when she became involved with the Collaboration, having worked with Australia's Consumers Health Forum and National Health and Medical Research Council. The Collaboration might have helped her to develop professionally through her exposure to the people in its orbit, but she was already grounded in the concept of bias when Iain Chalmers asked her to get involved.

Even before the Collaboration became an established entity, Bastian was using evidence to argue for change, especially around pregnancy and childbirth. She made frequent use of the two-volume *Effective Care in Pregnancy and Childbirth*, which she calls the "first giant set of reviews covering everything."

She makes it sound easy, how she used evidence to make points, to lobby for positions and to support women's rights around childbirth. She said of that early time, "I was a consumer advocate, and all I had to do before I went into a meeting would be to really study that particular chapter in the original two books." Which is to say, she wasn't an expert on the evidence but she knew where to find the best evidence.

She went on: "And if you boned up on those things, you could walk into a meeting with all of these obstetricians who would make various claims, and then say something like, 'Well... Smith in 1982 showed blah, blah, blah.' And then you could go, 'Well, yes, but Jones in 1985, said blah, blah, blah...'" She's quick to the point, adding that having the evidence gave her a huge leg-up as an effective bullshit detector. "You understood where they were claiming things as facts that were essentially totally untested theories." Having the evidence on hand, for her, "really changed everything."

She remembers the obvious paternalism at the beginning. Some people didn't think consumers needed to be involved. After all, in some quarters, consumers are considered "bias personified," said Bastian. Others said: "Look. I'm a person. I consume. I'm a patient too."

Bastian believes that the Collaboration, now past its 20-year mark, "doesn't necessarily have a lot of input coming in from many people outside. And there is a lot of co-option from a consumer's point of view." Which is to say that consumer representatives, over time, start to relate more and more to the needs of researchers and the academic reviewers, and become ever more removed from everyday consumers.

She says that for many consumers, "Cochrane is their primary involvement, or the only place at which they represent consumers. Many have other roles in health care, as clinicians or scientists, and it would be wrong to think of everyone as having a 'legitimate' consumer base."

She moderates that sentiment by saying, "The one thing to remember about Cochrane is that it's not one specific organization or one specific culture. It's like 50 separate little cultures, and it's different depending on which topic area you're interested in." In some groups, consumer input is welcomed and embraced, and the reviewers say, 'Thank heavens you've arrived. We've been waiting for you!'" she says, while with others, "You could never get any kind of foot in the door."

It also varies by culture. In some countries, the review authors find it difficult to form natural alliances with consumers, and some are paternalistic toward consumers. Bastian states that this doesn't seem to depend on how rich the country is, and she's seen both paternalism and an incredible openness to consumer input on all rungs of the development ladder.

What does Bastian consider the biggest challenge ahead? She told me, "I think it's still to create something that is more usable," which is a poignant remark from someone who has been summarizing the results of systematic reviews for more than 25 years.

She underlines this point by saying, "When the vast majority of people on the planet go looking for health information, they are not going to Cochrane reviews," and that the Collaboration's work is "still a thimble in an ocean."

There is a variety of reasons for the Collaboration's low profile

with the general public globally, but for Bastian, the explana-
tion that makes the most sense is that the "kind of questions
that people have, clinicians and patients, is not the way academia
structures its information." The information in systematic reviews
of evidence is not (in form or substance) something that makes
consumers beat a path to the Collaboration's door.

No one would deny that the Collaboration's outputs have to
be usable products – usable for all users of health research. They
have to be, Bastian says, "where people go for information; where
they need information; where they use information." She says
that it's futile to think that Cochrane will somehow "train the
entire planet to use information in a different way; ask questions
in a different way; go to a place they ordinarily wouldn't go." Her
biggest wish: "Instead of trying to adapt everybody on the planet
to Cochrane, working on how to adapt Cochrane more to the
planet."

Hilda Bastian was reflecting an attitude I heard from many
people inside and outside Cochrane, that the organization needed
to better reflect the needs of everyday people. That sentiment was
most notably emphasized by Iain Chalmers, in many of the actions he supported in setting up the original Collaboration and
in his subsequent work. When Chalmers retired from the UK
Cochrane Centre in 2002, he started the James Lind Initiative, a
programme funded by the National Institute for Health Research
to promote better research for better health care.

Chalmers has often noted the mismatch between what is of
interest to researchers versus what is most important to patients
and the clinicians to whom they look for help. In 1998 in the
BMJ he wrote that "greater public involvement could help to reduce this mismatch and ensure that trials are designed to address
questions that patients see as relevant."[88] While acknowledging
some progress in this area, he felt there was much more work to

do. The James Lind Alliance (www.lindalliance.org) has undoubt-edly become one of the most active and important vehicles for in-volving the users of health research in discussions about research, especially around identifying and prioritizing uncertainties.

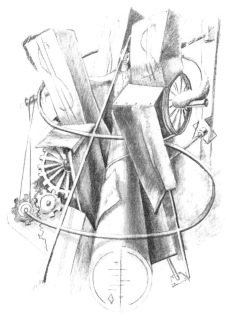

SEVEN

A Shining Light:
Drugs and Money

"Everything for me is marketing and publicity,
unless proven otherwise."

– Tom Jefferson

WHY WOULD one of the world's biggest drug companies listen to what some individual working in the Cochrane Collaboration says about them? After all, this drug company is an institution of immense wealth and power, able to withstand all kinds of rock-pelting and carry on perfectly well. It has a public relations department that can handle attacks from all comers, and annual revenues that eclipse many government health budgets. Why bother listening to a lone voice in the wilderness asking some un-comfortable questions?

Maybe it's because those questions expose the weaknesses of the evidence that underlies one of its most profitable products.

Tamiflu and Transparency

Back in 2003, the Swiss drug giant, Roche, published a trial showing the effectiveness of a drug that had been approved by the US Food and Drug Administration in 1997: the antiviral drug oseltamivir (known as Tamiflu). Dr. Tom Jefferson, known as the Collaboration's "flu guy," led a team interested in this drug and others promoted as preventing the spread of influenza.

To get to the bottom of what the drug could or couldn't do, Tom asked the trialists who had studied Tamiflu if they could supply the full unpublished dataset. They referred him to the trial sponsor – Roche – which had paid for the research. This was, perhaps, more than a subtle acknowledgement that those re-searchers had actually little control over their own data.

Jefferson wasn't just being a troublemaker. He was doing what he thought any good Cochrane review author must do: keep his review up to date. The review concerned a whole class of drugs known as neuraminidase inhibitors, prescribed to reduce the length and the severity of influenza symptoms. It was possible that new information from Roche could affect Jefferson's review. The implications could be huge. Tamiflu was one of the key drugs stockpiled by governments around the world to respond to a po-tential influenza pandemic.[89]

About a decade has passed – a decade that included prepara-tions for a worldwide influenza pandemic that never happened – and Jefferson has worked like a dog to get those missing data.

The value of the unpublished Tamiflu data increased con-siderably when, in June of 2009, the World Health Organization (WHO) declared a global influenza pandemic, invoking fears of a

1918-style influenza outbreak. Following the WHO's recommendations, the world's health systems accelerated their stockpiling
of Tamiflu, spending as much as $7 billion (US, in 2009 dollars)
over the next few years.

Fear of the flu was no doubt stoked by invoking the catas-
trophic 1918 influenza epidemic, one of the worst human health
disasters in history. About 500 million people around the world
were infected, and somewhere between 50 million and 100 million deaths resulted. Whether or not it was wise for the WHO
to recommend that nations around the world stockpile Tamiflu
remains an open question, but one thing is certain: no one was
really sure how well the drug would work to halt an epidemic,
or whether such expenditure could have financed more effective
measures in combating the spread of a pandemic flu virus.

In 2009, as the Collaboration's influenza researchers, notably Jefferson and his colleague Peter Doshi, were updating their
review, they got a surprise. They were contacted by a Japanese
pediatrician who alerted them to the presence of eight unpublished Tamiflu trials. As Jefferson later wrote, those studies
couldn't be included in his review update because he hadn't seen
the original studies.[90]

They wrote to the trialists and to the company, Roche, to ask
for the data and were rebuffed. This seemed like the tip of an ice-
berg because, as they dug, they discovered many more trials. The
list grew from 26 to 123 – and the vast majority of those trials
were Roche-sponsored. Jefferson and his team started to demand
some answers.

They began a letter-writing campaign explicitly asking Roche
for all of the data that had been used to demonstrate the effectiveness of Tamiflu. They reasoned that those data were vital to
assess the benefits and harms of the drug. Surely this information
needed to be out in the open, available for public scrutiny – all

the more so as the world's governments were so heavily investing in and depending on this one drug.

In December, 2010, following the publication of the Cochrane review – both in the *Cochrane Library* and the *BMJ* – the company agreed to hand over the data. The public outcry started to grow, fuelled both by media reports and the *BMJ*'s decision to launch an experiment in November, 2012. The *BMJ* began publishing correspondence between members of the Cochrane Collaboration and Roche, the US Centers for Disease Control, and the WHO. The *BMJ* had been following this case for years, initially publicizing the fight over data between the Collaboration and Roche back in 2009. Its willingness to publish the correspondence between the Cochrane authors, Roche, and these public health bodies attracted a lot of attention.

The web-published correspondence (available to anyone with an Internet connection at http://www.bmj.com/tamiflu) shows an at-times hilarious back-and-forth dialogue. Jefferson's rebuttals are works of perseverance and civility, and the answers he got back were largely ludicrous "dog-ate-my-data" excuses. In fact, the whole episode reminded me of a typical parliamentary exchange in Canada where the opposition critic asks specific, direct questions of government ministers, and the ministers strenuously avert answering the questions, choosing instead to fill airtime with defensive PR spin.

At one point, Roche offered Jefferson and colleagues the data – as long as they all signed confidentiality agreements. This they refused, reasoning that doing so would make it impossible for them to complete the work for which they had requested the data in the first place.

There were many questions swirling around Tamiflu, but the key one that Cochrane researchers wanted answered was this: How can we know if the drug works unless we can look at the entire dataset that the company collected when it tested the drug?

Notwithstanding the world's stockpiles of the drug, the pandemic fears, and energetic efforts to "do something" in response, this question remains urgently relevant. It seems elementary that health regulators around the world should know if the billions they spent on a single drug were invested well.

Even though Roche had handed over thousands of pages of data to Tom Jefferson and his colleagues (and claimed to have sent the complete data to the health regulators), there remained many questions. Jefferson knew that there were more than 100 trials of Tamiflu, yet more than half the patient data from those trials still remained unpublished. The *BMJ*'s editor, Fiona Godlee, recognized that if these trials remained unpublished, then the researchers' main concern, an "overstating of effectiveness and the apparent under-reporting of potentially serious adverse effects," was likely.[91]

What hasn't been said publicly, though Jefferson and colleagues continue to ask, is this: "What's with all the secrecy?" Their position seemed unequivocal: If you have nothing to hide, then hide nothing.

It should be understood that publishing trial results is not always under the control of researchers, and that the matter of making research data publicly available is multifaceted.

With the help of the *BMJ*'s Open Data project, the Collaboration has been able to increase the pressure, and not just on Roche. The WHO and the US Centers for Disease Control (CDC), which recommended Tamiflu as a way to stop the spread of influenza, are also on the hit list.

The WHO had put oseltamivir (Tamiflu) on its "essential drugs list" (a list of about 300 medications considered vital to treating the majority of the world's maladies). As Tom Jefferson suggested in the *BMJ*, a drug like oseltamivir, the effectiveness of which is still an open question, should not be in this small basket of proven, lifesaving medications, which includes drugs such as penicillin and insulin.

So why were Jefferson and colleagues also taking on the CDC? As he told the *BMJ*, "The CDC has extensively recommended the use of Tamiflu, and, as you know, governments worldwide have stockpiled it on the advice, essentially, of WHO." He added, "We were trying to find out exactly what evidence these decisions were made on. So we asked questions, and we also asked WHO and CDC whether they'd seen our review and what their thoughts were."[92]

On a more philosophical note, what's really at stake here is the fact that scientific progress doesn't *progress* when the science is kept secret. Secrecy is about commercial objectives – making money for patent holders, or defending government decisions. While some clinical trial researchers may see legitimate reasons for closely guarding research data – patient confidentiality, for example – most would agree that it's a serious issue when important health-related research data are kept from public scrutiny.

Fast forward to April 2014, where the *BMJ*'s International Editor Kamran Abassi essentially summed up the Tamiflu saga in a commentary entitled: "The missing data that cost $20 billion."[93] He writes: "This week is the culmination of a five-year campaign led by Jefferson's Cochrane research team, supported by the *BMJ*, to ensure the release of the full clinical trial data on neuraminidase inhibitors. The studies, analyses and editorials in this issue strike like a hammer blow." Noting that the manufacturer had managed to generate sales in excess of $18 billion (US) of Tamiflu, he added that "the revised Cochrane reviews, which were based on the full clinical trial data, conclude that the benefits of the drugs don't outweigh the harms."

I think the world owes a round of applause to pesky researchers such as Jefferson and his team, and initiatives such as the *BMJ*'s Open Data campaign fuelled by dogged determination to make sure the whole truth was accessible to all. Over the years as I watched this scandal unfold, I read all the back and forth letters, press reports and challenges to medical authorities and drug makers (which anyone can access at bmj.com/Tamiflu) and am left with huge admiration for the perseverance of Jefferson and his colleagues in challenging the abomination of data secrecy.

It Keeps Happening

If you were to think that Tom Jefferson's battle over data secrecy with Roche is an anomaly in the history of the Cochrane Collaboration, you'd be wrong. In fact, Cochrane researchers have been striving for research transparency for decades. One of Iain Chalmers' early signature statements (outlined in a paper in the *Journal of the American Medical Association* in 1990) was repeated almost verbatim more than 20 years later in reference to the Tamiflu affair. He wrote: "Substantial numbers of clinical trials are never reported in print, and among those that are, many are not reported in sufficient detail to enable judgements to be made about the validity of their results. Failure to publish an adequate account of a well-designed clinical trial is a form of scientific misconduct that can lead those caring for patients to make inappropriate treatment decisions."[94]

In 2006, Chalmers himself weighed into the Tamiflu affair, writing a letter to John Bell, a Roche board member, and expressing his concern that it wasn't just scientific misconduct at stake in the Tamiflu affair, but also the public's trust in people holding positions of authority in health matters. Chalmers' message was clear: "Biased under-reporting of research is one of the factors jeopardizing public trust in biomedical research."[95]

When drug companies and regulators stifle debate and won't deal head on with serious concerns raised by researchers such as Tom Jefferson, science, and in this case, medical progress affecting everyone everywhere, is compromised. In November,

2012, Jefferson could have been summing up a *raison d'être* for the Cochrane Collaboration when he wrote to Roche for the umpteenth time, explaining "for the purposes of our research, we remain interested in conducting the most rigorous, independent assessment of Tamiflu that is possible, and remain interested in obtaining the full study reports promised in December, 2009 and complete de-identified electronic patient-level data."[96]

The most important word in that letter is "independent." The fight to keep the Collaboration independent is a story in itself.

Avoiding Bias: More Truths Can Come Out

Clive Adams is a psychiatrist who originally hails from Northern Ireland. When he speaks in a light Irish lilt, he exudes a mind filled with humor. For a guy who works around some of human-kind's most destructive diseases – those of the human mind such as schizophrenia and psychosis – he comes across as someone who finds much in the world immensely amusing. Adams founded the Cochrane Schizophrenia Group while at Oxford. He now lives in Nottingham, and 20 years on, continues as the group's co-ordinating editor.

I spoke with him in Madrid at the Cochrane Colloquium in 2011, and asked him what kind of changes he's seen since the early 1990s. He told me, "Some 20 years ago, when the Cochrane Collaboration was starting up, largely, the guidance for the care of people with schizophrenia was from well-meaning, very knowledgeable people who overviewed the literature in a traditional way and probably often got it right through wisdom and experience and their background knowledge. But you couldn't tell they were right, and it certainly was not science. What has happened since then is a remarkable investment in dragging science back into the process of reviewing, whereby you get much clearer answers, but also, you shine a light... as to whether the emperor is or is not wearing clothes."

He adds, referring to psychiatry, "I think my specialty more than others has wanted to be duped by the lack of knowledge, by the pharmaceutical industry – people with vested interests and psychological therapies – to feel that we have more powerful interventions than we really have, or more powerful data." He points out that the work of the Collaboration provides a systematic way to sort those data, adding that "the schizophrenia evidence has gone from being a chaotic sea of evidence to being much more ordered... and now it's gone through into many major guidelines."

I ask the "So what" question: Does Adams think that schizophrenics get better treatment now compared to 20 years ago? "Absolutely! Yes," he answers. "It has a huge journey yet to go – enormous – but what didn't used to be there is accessible evidence that can be used either by policymakers or by people with schizophrenia themselves. Or the clinicians, the busy clinician, and now those stakeholders all have much less excuse than they did have 20 years ago to at least have the evidence to go to."

He reminds me that the spread of this ordered evidence can help many of those who, perhaps, up to now have been left out by the advance in science and methods of systematic reviews. He said, "That in [2010], the WHO commissioned us to produce vast amounts of data for them because 80 percent of the world's population with schizophrenia lives in lower-income countries, so they wanted to know about the inexpensive interventions and the evidence behind them."

WHO Pays?

Having the WHO not only ask Cochrane researchers to help with systematic reviews but also provide funds to do those reviews raises an important point discussed from the earliest days of the Collaboration: how to fund the work of the Cochrane Collaboration.

From the Collaboration's earliest days, when the organization was a small band of founding members united by a shared vision, there has been much discussion and contentious debate about how the Collaboration should finance its activities. Part of that debate is about whether or not it would be appropriate for the Collaboration to accept money – any of it – from the pharmaceutical industry. Certainly, doing so would raise concerns about its reputation. The majority of the Collaboration's members and supporters maintain that drug industry funding would bias the Collaboration and ruin its reputation.

This issue affects all of medicine. Yet, the one medical specialty that has probably the strongest ties to the pharmaceutical industry is psychiatry – Clive Adams' area. In a famous editorial from 2000 ("Is Academic Medicine for Sale?[97]") Marcia Angell, the former editor of the *New England Journal of Medicine*, chose psychiatry as the specialty most beholden to drug companies. She admitted that when the *NEJM* was seeking independent US psychiatrists to write review articles about antidepressants, few could be found who were free from financial ties to drug manufacturers.

Adams himself states, "It is easy to bring up the pharmaceutical industry as a source of major bias in our area, and surely it is. And it may be a source of major bias where we, collectively, willingly lay ourselves open to being vulnerable to being influenced."

"However," he adds, "it is a relatively simple bias. The pharmaceutical industry – love them or hate them – are pretty well entirely predictable. How can you not be biased when $2 billion rests on the outcome in your studies?"

He certainly doesn't think that all pharmaceutical-funded studies should be thrown out, because "even despite that... more truths can come out of those studies and they can be fruitfully used within systematic reviews."

Adams says that it's not just the pharmaceutical industry that has biases. He reminds me of the biases of those promoting their own brands of psychological interventions or medical devices. Those who are invested in developing a treatment or intervention are naturally going to see it in the best possible light. The solution? "I think we are riven with bias, but part of what Cochrane can do is to dispassionately shine a light on that; and that, in itself, slowly has [changed] and will change the culture."

Pay the Piper, Call the Tune

Peter Gøtzsche, head of the Nordic Cochrane Centre, told me that his experiences with the pharmaceutical industry have hardened his mettle over the years.[98]

He recalls a time when he was publicly taken to task after publishing a study on academic freedom. He had said that, if a drug company sponsors a trial, it owns the data and it needs to approve the manuscript and so on. Essentially such an arrangement means that "academic freedom is almost non-existent." After he published that study, the Danish association of the pharmaceutical industry accused him and his team of scientific misconduct.

He continues, "I was so furious about this because, of course, we hadn't committed scientific misconduct. It was pure harassment." The story eventually came out in the *BMJ*.

Gøtzsche was later part of a team comparing pairs of meta-analyses (published within two years of each other) that looked at the use of two particular drugs in treating a particular disease. The team examined 24 meta-analyses that matched Cochrane reviews. One-third were industry-supported, one-third had undeclared support, and one-third had no support or were supported by non-industry sources.

The results: "Compared with industry-supported reviews and reviews with undeclared support, Cochrane reviews had more often considered the potential for bias in the review." While this article generated considerable debate within the pages of the *BMJ*, the conclusion that "industry-supported reviews of drugs should be read with caution," was a fairly secure take-home message. Gøtzsche's conclusions were that the industry-supported studies were "less transparent, had few reservations about methodological limitations of the included trials, and had more favorable conclusions than the corresponding Cochrane reviews."[99]

It seems as if, as time goes on, Peter Gøtzsche's criticism of biased research is getting more shrill. He tells me that we have to be scrupulous in minimizing bias, especially when it comes to drug treatments, because the treatments could be immensely harmful. He adds, "We know too little about them, particularly because the drug industry hides the harms of their treatments. We want to have that out in the open."

Industry Funding: a Contentious Issue

It was early October, 1999, and the seventh Cochrane Colloquium was set to take place at the Università S. Tomaso D'Aquino, in the heart of Rome. Many of the delegates were delighted to be invited to the city, with its world class museums and the Coliseum – a site so soaked in history that it is designated by UNESCO as a World Heritage Site. Most of the meeting rooms were in the seventeenth century cloister, next to the main hall and surrounded by magnificent gardens facing the Roman forum.

Rome is significant in Cochrane history because it was here, in this ancient capital, that one of the more contentious issues in the Collaboration's history began to be debated.

At this meeting, Lisa Bero, a professor of pharmacy and health policy at the University of California in San Francisco and a long-time Collaboration member, was asked to chair a debate on the topic of industry funding within the organization.

Funding has been discussed ever since the Collaboration began, and the dominant view among participants seemed to be that if the pharmaceutical industry were allowed to fund the creation of reviews, the Collaboration risked producing tainted and biased information. At the very least, the perception of taking money from industry could reflect poorly on the independence of the organization and its credibility.

Bero was the right person to chair such a debate. An experienced Cochrane contributor, she understood the issues deeply. She was also among a handful of researchers there who had produced original research on the influence of industry funding on research. She had published papers showing that such influence affects the design, conduct and publication of research in ways that introduce bias towards that industry's products. With her depth of knowledge on the issue, she was well equipped to steer this discussion in a productive direction.[100]

Bero has been involved with the Collaboration almost from the beginning, on the urging of one of her mentors, Dr. Drummond Rennie. Rennie is long-time Deputy Editor of the *Journal of the American Medical Association*, and it was he who introduced Bero to the Collaboration. Bero recalls Rennie telling her, "Look, Lisa. It won't make you rich or advance your career, but you have to get to know these people. They are some of the smartest people around and they are *very* interested in finding out what works."

Bero has more than just a passing interest in what works. For her, the Cochrane Collaboration was a natural fit, since a large portion of the evidence being systematized and analyzed by Cochrane contributors involved drug treatments. She became interested because of the methods, but perhaps it was her stronger interest in how that evidence was used in policy-making that made her devote her energies to studying bias.

The debate in Rome that October was organized by the conference head, the late Alessandro Liberati, and featured a panel of Italian academics, researchers, and some people who worked with the industry. The Collaboration's leadership was drafting a commercial sponsorship policy at the time, and they believed that hashing it out in the Colloquium would help air the various perspectives on the question of industry funding.

Chairing the debate was a delicate task. Bero, who is passionate about the topic herself and known for being "a blunt American," remembers that, before the debate, she got a gentle warning from Liberati. He told her, "Lisa, you are in Italy and you can't cut people off. You have to let people speak."

On this topic, Liberati understood how important it was to have both sides air their views. Some in the Italian medical community were keen to allow Cochrane activities to be funded by the pharmaceutical industry, though Liberati himself would not have held that view. Bero remembers the discussion as heated, at times volatile, but vital. She called it "the turning point for the sponsorship debate."

The results of this discussion formed the basis of a draft commercial sponsorship policy. Bero, as a member of the Steering Group at the time, did a lot of the drafting. It was sent out for comments, and Bero remembers, "We got a ton of comments back, which the committee collated and analyzed and used to modify the proposed policy."

The policy at its heart was relatively simple. Individual Cochrane reviews could not be funded by the manufacturer of a drug or other product discussed in those reviews. The question of funding for centres or methods groups was not as clearly defined in this initial policy.

As the years rolled on, the debate continued. In Stavanger, Norway, in 2002, Ron Koretz remembers one particular business meeting where the issue at hand was whether the Collaboration would allow corporations to sponsor the organization's annual conferences (colloquia)[101].

What could be more innocuous than having a few

corporations supply funding so that the Collaboration could have a good meeting once a year? Koretz recalls, "At that time, the Steering [Group] put forth a policy that, under certain circumstances, the Collaboration would accept donations from industry [to support colloquia]. A number of people in the audience, including myself, went to the microphone to protest such a move. I feared that we would lose credibility… and that this would become the first step down a very slippery slope."

That discussion was a small affair compared to what happened the next year, in Barcelona. Then, the issue was debated at the opening plenary session and at a series of other meetings. The goal was to get comments from the participants to develop another consultation document that could be circulated. These things don't generally happen in a hurry. The process of reforming the policy demonstrated the Collaboration's egalitarian, democratic processes. What happened was captured in a *BMJ* article by Australian journalist Ray Moynihan: "Cochrane at Crossroads over Drug Company Sponsorship."[102]

Moynihan summarized the events in Barcelona in a lengthy article drawn from interviews with those who held strong opinions on opposite sides of the debate. He mapped out the arguments put forth by the opponents of pharma funding, citing the perception and risks of biases, and the views of proponents, who said that industry funding could make the Collaboration's activities more sustainable. In his conclusion, he foreshadowed another debate that the Collaboration has since had to contend with. This he described as "the even more difficult question of the individual financial ties of researchers who produce Cochrane reviews."

He highlighted the nub of the issue, which goes beyond Cochrane and affects any medical matter in which issues of conflicts of interest arise: "The delegates at Barcelona can take some small comfort from knowing they are by no means alone. Indeed, they will generate considerable global interest if they can design a foolproof mechanism for accepting sponsorship and ensuring independence."[103]

Toward Evidence-Based Internal Policy

Jim Neilson, the editor of the Pregnancy and Childbirth Group, was one of the co-chairs of the Steering Group at the Barcelona Colloquium in 2003. It was his task to chair the Collaboration's Annual General Meeting – including the open question and discussion session.[104]

He described the meeting in Barcelona in one word: "Pain." This wasn't just referring to the discussions about the commercial sponsorship policy; it was also because poor Jim himself was in pain. He said, "My main recollection of Barcelona was having a dental abscess, involving several days without sleep… so I struggled a bit there."

He admits that it was a struggle in formulating an acceptable policy, which "was something that took a little bit of time to resolve completely so everyone was on board with it."

For context, Neilson told me that, at that time, "it was pretty difficult to get funding. We were pretty lucky in the UK. Our review groups are funded mostly by the National Health Service. But for other countries, it was difficult to get infrastructure funding – and that did have implications for groups doing a good job under difficult circumstances."

At the same time, he said, there was "a pretty clear view from most people in the Collaboration that there shouldn't be any direct sponsorship of systematic reviews by commercial entities that stood to gain from the findings of the review. I think everyone was on board with that."

The complexity involved some activities of the Collaboration that were somewhat removed from the development of systematic reviews. There were the translation initiatives – specifically, translating reviews into Spanish – which were really important, not only for Spain, but also for Latin America, and which were funded by commercial entities.

Neilson: "It was a concern that some groups would go under. But everybody felt the policy of funding reviews and review groups was pretty clear-cut, and if an entity went under, it was unfortunate, but that was the cost that had to be paid."

The battle in Barcelona was, by all reports, intense. Peter Gøtzsche said, "It wasn't really nice because... emotions were running high, and we weren't always very popular when we fought against industry funding of Cochrane activities."

Lisa Bero came away with an indelible insight from that meeting: "What struck me was that Cochrane collaborators, who are ALL about the evidence, can conveniently ignore the evidence about biases introduced by industry funding! The issue is not pure emotion. We have evidence!"

The Barcelona debate on this issue became more surreal in the rumor mill. Jini Hetherington recalled, "A rumor had been circulating that the Steering Group was going to open up the Collaboration to industry funding. So the questions from the floor were pointed and direct." The problem was, there were no grounds for such rumor, and the members of the Steering Group sat by, a bit bemused, listening to speaker after passionate speaker coming to the microphone with strong questions and harsh criticisms.

"It didn't help," Hetherington noted, "that Jim Neilson was sitting through this in intense pain."

In early 2004, the Steering Group held a meeting and revised the policy, keeping in place the prohibition on industry funding of reviews. Funding policies for other activities, such as for centres and methods groups, have since been tightened. Today, one actually sees very little overt pharmaceutical industry activity at colloquia or supporting the Collaboration's work. As this book goes to press, the Collaboration is carrying out further revisions to its policies concerning sponsorship. Funding challenges remain, however. As Peter Gøtzsche explains, "The workload of Cochrane review groups increases exponentially. It is untenable, and we just need more funding for the Cochrane review groups." But should that money come from industry? "No," he says, "It should come from governments." In his opinion, if the organization needs pharma money to survive, "Well then, the Cochrane Collaboration shouldn't survive. It should stop... because there is so much research that shows that when you start getting industry money, you start getting undue influence."

Disclosure of Funding: Where and How

There is another chapter in the story concerning the way in which the pharmaceutical industry could affect the Collaboration's work. What if most of the studies in a review are industry-funded studies, which have a tendency to favor the drugs studied? Should that be disclosed as a routine part of a Cochrane review?

Several people raised this issue within the Collaboration, including New York consumer-health activist Maryann Napoli, who believe that people need to know who paid for the studies under review. It concerns her that the part of a Cochrane review most likely to be read by consumers – the summary, or abstract —is incomplete without a disclosure of funding sources. One solution might be that people should read the full reviews, but the reviews themselves sometimes don't disclose this information.

Michelle Roseman, a master's student at McGill University in Montreal, was the lead author on two *BMJ* articles (from 2011 and 2012) that examine the question of funding disclosure. Her team of researchers, which included Lisa Bero, found that "funding sources for studies included in Cochrane reviews are rarely reported (in RoB [risk of bias] tables or included studies tables)."[105]

Bero reminded me that "funding source" is still not recognized as a risk of bias in *The Cochrane Handbook for Systematic Reviews of Interventions*, the Collaboration's principal resource for the preparation of systematic reviews.[106]

The funding issue is not as simple as it might seem. Some researchers within the Collaboration feel not only that disclosure of clinical trial funding is already adequately dealt with in Cochrane reviews, but also that the reviews themselves are shaped to uncover the most important biases (how the study was designed, how blinding occurred, etc.) which makes disclosing financial conflicts moot.

Bero would counter this sentiment, saying, "When we control for those other sources of bias, we still see a bias that is related to *funding* bias." She also points out, "Everyone has a common goal of producing high-quality work. It's part of who we are. It's not taking someone's word for anything." She emphasizes, "We are not asking Cochrane [authors] to ignore industry-funded trials… We just want Cochrane reviews to be transparent about how much their findings depend on industry-funded trials and to recognize that there are biases associated with this funding."

Obviously, this is one of those debates that will continue for some time and, for me, underscores a few notable points about the Cochrane Collaboration. It shows the organization's ability to be self-critical, to indicate where it might be failing, and its willingness to nudge itself into improvements. Bero told me, with a chuckle in her voice, "It's a very self-critical organization – the most navel-gazing organization I've ever seen." She's probably not alone in that sentiment.

Moreover, you don't suggest changes in the Collaboration unless you can first come up with evidence for why change should occur. If Bero stood up and said, "Cochrane reviews don't reveal financial conflicts of included studies (and that's a bad thing)," she would risk being challenged with something like, "Sure, Lisa. I hope you have some evidence to convince us." She does.

If you have a strong opinion, you'd better make sure that you have an evidence basis for it. That's the Cochrane way. And many Cochrane members wouldn't change such a momentous internal policy about who may fund its activities unless it was working from a decent evidence base and allowed a full airing of various viewpoints.

This story continues, and it may be a while before it's fully resolved, if ever. Passionate arguments will continue. People will continue to debate the effects of such policies. Above all, in the heated debates of the future, people in the Collaboration will come back to that perennial question: "What does the evidence say?" That's the Cochrane way.

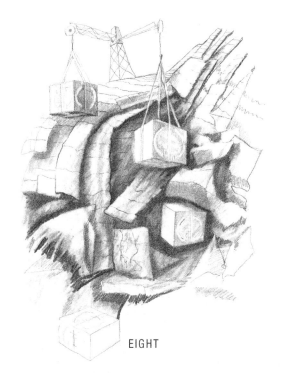

EIGHT

Cochrane and Disaster Response: Evidence Aid

---

*"The conscience of the world is so guilty
that it always assumes that those
who investigate heresies must be heretics."*

— Aleister Crowley

AS PEOPLE in Europe were waking up on December 26, 2004, their minds might not have been focused on charity, or thinking about what they could do for their fellow humans. They soon would be. The news that greeted people that morning, first with a trickle, then a flood, described a massive undersea earthquake off the coast of Indonesia, triggering a tsunami of near-apocalyptic proportions.

Centered off the coast of Sumatra, the tsunami rolled ashore without warning. Waves as high as 30 meters – a steamroller of destruction – killed an estimated 230,000 people in 14 countries, and left millions more homeless and displaced in an arc bordering the Indian Ocean. The destruction was most acute in the countries near the epicenter: Indonesia, India, Sri Lanka and Thailand. The scale of this natural disaster, and of the megathrust earthquake that triggered it, was one of the largest in recorded history. The energy released by the shifting of deep undersea tectonic plates was more than 1,500 times that of the Hiroshima atomic bomb. So large, in fact, that scientists have said that it caused the planet to wobble on its axis.

A natural disaster of this scale, with the massive loss of life and immense destruction it entailed, draws all of us – the world's bystanders – to the calamity. And it makes many of us ask: What can we do to alleviate the suffering, and how can we help deliver that aid as fast as possible?

Assessing Interventions

Those living in the awareness of Archie Cochrane's mindset may ask more nuanced questions. In the rush to deliver immediate, large-scale, and urgently needed aid, is it possible that this deeply felt humanitarian impulse could lead us astray? Is it possible that our philanthropy could leave people worse off? Such questions are almost never voiced; certainly not in the panic of the moment or the adrenaline-fuelled rush to help in whatever manner possible – at least not in a systematic way.

But those questions were swirling through the minds of people in the Cochrane Collaboration – people such as Mike Clarke, who had recently ended his term as chair of the Collaboration's Steering Group and was director of the UK

Cochrane Centre in Oxford. He had witnessed the utter devastation on his TV and was as eager as anyone to help. As a long-time researcher, he would also ask: If we want to deliver aid, what kind of aid? What's the best way to do it? Is there a good evidence base supporting the kinds of humanitarian relief being sent to the survivors? Is it possible that people could be harmed by interventions designed to help? If monetary aid is insufficient to meet the scale of suffering, what's the most efficient way to deliver an emergency response that wrings the most aid possible out of each donor's dollar?[107]

Clarke has worked assessing both actions and interventions in health care for most of his professional life. Now based at Queen's University in Belfast, he is not yet well known for his work in humanitarian circles, but he has worked hard to try to improve the accessibility of Cochrane reviews in low- and middle-income countries. He spent much of his time as a student at the University of Oxford working in a shelter for homeless people. He is also one of the Collaboration's go-to people for designing trials that capture what they need to capture.

Together with colleagues from around the world, Clarke has worked on a variety of large randomized trials in diverse fields such as maternity care, breast cancer, poisoning, and stroke. He has helped in preparing more than 30 systematic reviews of even wider diversity: from the effects of flight socks to ways to improve response to postal questionnaires, the scale of publication bias, and the effect of salary increases on civil servants in low-income countries.

Clarke watched the devastation unfold in southeast Asia. On a blog called *Cochrane Gems* he wrote (under a pseudonym):

What can we do? Aid needs evidence on what works and what doesn't work. It is no good and, worse, might be harmful, to deliver health care that is ineffective. Those of us who work in the production of evidence can, therefore, deliver our own form of aid: information. The provision of reliable information on the effects of health care is the way that many of us can contribute to alleviating its effects. We need to recognize the privileged position that we are in: we can help by doing what we do best.[108]

He was not alone in his desire to use Cochrane evidence to help. As he described it in an article written with Prathap Tharyan and Sally Green, published in *PLOS Medicine* in June, 2005: "Shortly after the tsunami, it was felt that the Cochrane Collaboration, as the world's largest international organization committed to providing good evidence about health care, and with many members working in the region, had a moral duty to help in the global relief and rehabilitation efforts."[109]

Luckily, the Collaboration already had a network of people around the world gathering evidence on infectious diseases, water quality, injury management, and other immediate health care needs associated with natural disasters. With people at WHO, that small working group drew up a list of more than "200 interventions considered relevant to health care in the aftermath of the tsunami," and set out to prioritize and group them according to criteria such as whether or not current reviews were available or needed to be updated or created.

As part of this effort, the *Cochrane Library's* publisher, John Wiley & Sons, agreed to provide free, one-click access to everyone in the affected countries for a six-month period, from February to July, 2005. Clarke remembers that Clive Adams, from the Cochrane Schizophrenia Group, stressed the need to take the information in Cochrane reviews and make it free to people confronted by the tsunami's aftermath. They agreed that this was the right thing to do. Soon government and healthcare agencies carrying out health planning and relief efforts received unlimited access to *The Cochrane Library*.

Bias Affects Even Disaster Response

Bonnix Kayabu, a young doctor from the Democratic Republic of Congo, has seen his share of humanitarian crises. He has worked in the Congo and in Rwanda and went to Ireland to study. When interviewed in 2011, he was one of the Collaboration's newer members.[110]

Kayabu said that he first encountered the Collaboration in 2009, while working toward his master's degree in global health at Trinity College in Dublin: "There was a module called 'Introduction to systematic reviews.' Mike Clarke, who was the director of the UK Cochrane Centre, taught one of these modules, and I found it very interesting."

Just after finishing his master's degree, Kayabu learned that Clarke was thinking about how to formalize the collection of evidence for humanitarian crises. After the Haiti earthquake of January, 2010, and as part of a program supported by the Cochrane Collaboration for funding to take Evidence Aid to a new level, Clarke approached him for help.

According to Clarke, Evidence Aid could either continue as a response mechanism, deployed whenever a major disaster struck, or it could be built into a permanent, accessible resource for reducing the risk of future disasters and for planning, response and recovery. In either case, it had a future that they could shape in accord with Cochrane principles.

The Collaboration and John Wiley & Sons gave Evidence Aid some initial funding to support the appointment of a coordinator. Clarke asked Kayabu to take on this role, to work with aid agencies, NGOs, and others involved in the humanitarian response to disasters. Kayabu's initial task would be to identify their needs and determine how to meet them with an Evidence Aid website and database.

When I interviewed him, Kayabu was frank about the challenges that faced Evidence Aid. He said, "There are many types of evidence, but scientific evidence in the area of humanitarian work was poor and we knew it. Research that we managed to find proved that the evidence was poor."

Kayabu initiated a "bottom-up" research strategy, starting with the people on the receiving end of evidence – mostly administrators and humanitarian and emergency-relief organizations. What did they need? What was lacking? When did they need information: before, during, or after natural disasters and other complex emergencies?

Simply, Kayabu wanted to find out what were the most important needs for systematic reviews, the gaps in the evidence base, and what kinds of information (such as guidelines from health ministries in the country where they work) were guiding the efforts of humanitarian organizations.

Kayabu is well aware of the bias that can influence professionals who "have their own unique way of seeing a medical problem, delivering a diagnosis, and treating." And there are not just biases toward certain types of medicines; there are also biases shaping how we respond to healthcare crises, and the kind of evidence that develops around those responses.

It's clear that the 2004 tsunami deeply affected the mental health of its survivors. Many people who survived the tragedy had physical injuries, but even those who escaped physical harm were afflicted by depression, anxiety, and worse.

When the horror of the tsunami became known, there was a strong need, driven by heavy media pressure and the push by local administrations, to "do something." After providing burial, first aid, and other immediate medical care to survivors, the greatest need was for psychological interventions to deal with the mental trauma experienced by survivors. Survivor guilt and remorse, in addition to post-traumatic stress disorder (PTSD), were evident.

One proposal to help these people was to provide a single debriefing session to groups in each village. The thinking was that this would be efficient and provide comprehensive coverage. Another was to identify those considered at risk of developing long-term problems, and then to provide supportive care and follow-up for them. Of course, humans since the dawn of time have developed their own social and cultural norms around coping with disasters. Given their own inherent coping skills, the big question was: What was the right thing to do in the face of this enormous tragedy?

A Kind of Infection

April 1, 2002: Prathap Tharyan thought he'd received a scam e-mail. He deleted it.

The professor of psychiatry at the Christian Medical College, in Vellore, Tamil Nadu, India, is not easily fooled.[111] He said that the e-mail came from somebody who called himself a WHO consultant working with the Cochrane Collaboration and he told me: "I had never heard of the guy, but the email told me I'd just won a prize." He was told that it was the Kenneth Warren Prize, an award given out at the Colloquium every year to a member of the Collaboration from a developing country who had published a Cochrane review considered to be of high quality, on a topic relevant to health problems facing people in developing countries.

When you know whom the prize is named for, it gives it a bit of resonance and by all accounts, Dr. Kenneth Warren was a remarkable individual. He was a physician and medical pioneer whose contribution to health in developing countries was immense. He worked hard to draw attention to the "great neglected diseases," the huge killers that afflict a large proportion of the world's population; mostly infectious diseases and those caused primarily by parasites, poor water quality, and poor sanitation. He was known for his research into schistosomiasis, a parasitic disease transmitted by worms that contributes to anemia and malnutrition. The fact that this award was created (and given for the first time at the first Colloquium held in a low- or middle-income country, South Africa, in 2000) indicates how important it is to the Collaboration to recognize work in the developing world, where the need for evidence is particularly challenging.

Tharyan said, "I'd never heard of the Kenneth Warren Prize, and because it was the first of April – April Fools' Day – I didn't believe it. I thought it was a scam."

But it wasn't a scam. A little while later, Jini Hetherington stepped in, sending him an e-mail confirming it: "Prathap, you did actually win, and your prize is a free ticket and $1,000 US to go to the Colloquium in Stavanger, in Norway."

Tharyan recalls that Stavanger was his first and probably his most memorable Colloquium. He said, "A funny incident occurred. On that day, I was awarded the Kenneth Warren Prize, and because I was so grateful to the Collaboration for funding my ticket and introducing me to all of these people, I sang a song at the song contest. And I won the song contest!"

This event is known as the Collaboro-vision Song Contest, based on the Eurovision Song Contest, an annual affair in Europe perhaps made most famous when a young Swedish group named ABBA won in 1974 with a preposterous song called "Waterloo."

Tharyan remembers that competition in the Collaboro-vision Contest was fierce. His biggest contender that night was none other than an "ABBA look-alike group of pretty girls" who sang an adapted version of "Waterloo" (which they called "Your Review"). Cheesy but true. By all accounts, the dance floor was stuffed with colloquium delegates as Tharyan delivered a dazzling version of the 1991 hit "Losing my Religion" by the American rock group REM. Tharyan's version, featuring references to the gods Thor, Odin and Sackett, wowed the crowd.

The next day at the airport, as Prathap was getting ready to leave, many people recognized him. They universally said, "Hey, you're the guy who sang the song." He smiles broadly at the humor in it all. "Nobody remembered I'd won the Kenneth Warren Prize!"

Interestingly, for someone who lives in a country where infectious diseases are rampant, he refers to his introduction to the Collaboration as a kind of "infection" that he has seen spread from person to person. One of the early people who lured him into the Collaboration was psychiatrist Clive Adams. Tharyan says, waving his finger, a hint of mockery in his voice, "Clive Adams was the one. He was one of the founding editors of the Schizophrenia Group, and he infected me with this Cochrane bug. It's all his fault."

Now more than 20 years later, Tharyan has played a critical role in bringing the Collaboration's work to the second most populated nation on earth. He has collaborated on many systematic reviews in the fields of schizophrenia, infectious diseases, pain and palliative care, and acute respiratory infections, adopting the perspective of someone who has found a useful tool and wants to use it everywhere. He says, "It's a fever that I can't get rid of. But I'm happy I've got this illness. I want to spread it to everybody. Anyone who comes into contact with me. And I don't care what methods [I] use. I think it's one of the most important things I'm doing in my life."

As someone from a part of the world where many people have limited access to social and medical services, expensive drugs and other health technologies that those in richer countries take for granted, Tharyan found proof in the tsunami of how useful Cochrane evidence could be to many people in his life.

When Professional Help is an Inferior Substitute

Like it or not, we increasingly live in a world that tends to outsource the unpleasant tasks, such as dealing with death and tragedy.

In his 1995 book, *The Careless Society: Community and Its*

Counterfeits, American educator John L. McKnight contends that the modern tendency toward "professionalized services" has destroyed the very communities those services were designed to help. He writes that many societies are losing the resourcefulness to deal with their own problems. They fail to draw on and develop the talents and skills of their citizens.[112]

In many industrialized countries, social and medical services have been highly professionalized. In North America, for example, when there is a sudden tragedy, such as children killed in a school shooting spree, the response of authorities is predictable. They deploy teams of grief counselors. McKnight calls these kinds of services "counterfeits" – phony in that they usurp the inherent abilities and skills we all possess to make our way through the tough spots and tragedies in our lives; phony in that they may leave us worse off.

Any intervention able to do good can also do harm, and there is some evidence that "grief therapy" – the kind of counseling delivered by platoons of therapists brought in after a mass tragedy – may turn normal bereavement into something more pathological and, ultimately, not help those grieving. Those delivering the counseling, and the authorities who send them in, would claim that their services provide real benefit and insist that the support makes people better.

What would a Cochranite say? "That's all good, but where's your evidence?"

After the 2004 tsunami, large numbers of counselors were rushed to the affected areas to debrief the survivors. The debriefings were often, as described above, single sessions with large groups of people, after which the counselors would "rush on to the next tsunami-affected villages in the district." Prathap Tharyan said that this was the official response of the government, fuelled by media pressure and speculations that tsunami survivors needed counseling to avert PTSD.

Nonetheless, Tharyan's reading of the literature suggests that this approach was not wise. If the goal of debriefing was to reduce the extent of the survivors' psychological stress and to prevent them from developing PTSD, maybe it shouldn't be done. At all. He didn't have to go far to find some relevant literature in a Cochrane review on debriefing for people who have experienced trauma.[113]

Tharyan, writing with Mike Clarke and Sally Green, makes these points in a June, 2005 article in *PLOS*:

Well-meaning but misdirected and sometimes harmful interventions could be prevented if those making decisions about the nature of responses had access to reliable and up-to-date evidence of what works and what does not... Good-quality systematic reviews form the basis on which interventions should be implemented and on which new interventions should be planned and evaluated.[114]

When he lectured at the second Evidence Aid conference in Brussels in October, 2012, Tharyan spoke of further research that he had carried out surrounding the debriefing episodes, using focus groups held with survivors of the 2004 tsunami. Those focus groups revealed deeper meanings about how people actually rebuilt their lives; about the "societal changes and collective coping" that happened in the catastrophe's aftermath.

Some people were able to look past it as they rebuilt their lives, using positive attitudes, spiritual coping, and changes in community structures, which can really make an incredible difference. As one survivor said, "People in the neighboring towns forgot their communal and religious differences. They all came together to feed us, even before we asked them. We are so grateful! When we first returned to sea after [the] tsunami, we dedicated our first catch to them!"

Many of these people had experienced multiple losses and were still grieving deeply; but in Tharyan's observation, "Coping mechanisms exist at individual and community levels that enhance resilience in the face of adversity and enable normal functioning in the majority of those affected, without requiring professional intervention."

Undoubtedly, disasters transform people, in both positive and negative ways. Tharyan's opinion: "Disaster relief efforts should facilitate, and not impede or delay, such transformations."

Tharyan says that evidence in medicine is important, but it's also a "two-edged sword." Theories only go so far, and it is what happens under real-world conditions that matters. He explains, "First you get the evidence right; make sure it works against no treatment or an alternative treatment. Then you ask, 'How does it work with what I would normally do?'"

Sometimes research happens in such rarefied conditions that applying results to a real-world setting is impossible. As Muir Gray explained to me: it is all about "relating efficacy shown in randomized controlled trials to effectiveness – namely, how will [any medical intervention] work in Middlesbrough or Gary, Indiana, on a wet Thursday afternoon."

To which I'd add, how will this health intervention work in Tamil Nadu province after the most devastating tsunami in modern history?

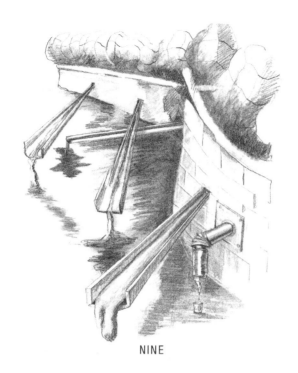

NINE

Gold-Standard Evidence:
Why National Healthcare Systems
Need Cochrane

---

*"Part of what we want to do is to make sure that those
decisions are being made by doctors and medical experts
based on evidence, based on what works, because
that's not how it's working right now."*

— US President Barack Obama, July 22, 2009

A REPORT released in September, 2012 in the United States contained some alarming figures. It said that about one-third of the money spent on US health care – about US$750 billion every year – was wasted. *Wasted.*

One could point to many ironies about health care, but probably one of the cruelest is that the USA, one of the richest countries in the world, funds the world's most expensive health care, but it's clearly getting ripped off, as the health of its population is among the poorest in the industrialized world. Americans spend a lot and get little for it – a situation that wastes in excess of US$2 billion per day on useless, untested, or inappropriate care. The report *Best Care at Lower Cost: The Path to Continuously Learning Health Care in America*[115] says that approximately 75,000 deaths could be averted each year if every US state delivered care at the same quality level as the best-performing state.

These facts are hard to swallow for Americans who believe that their healthcare system is the most advanced in the world, employs the highest of the high tech, and is almost always the early adopter of new technology, from drugs to robotic surgeons to gene therapies. Yet many families in the USA live in anxiety, a heartbeat or a tumor away from personal bankruptcy.

Excessive spending on the overuse and inappropriate use of health care threatens to bankrupt national, state, and family budgets. Journalist Shannon Brownlee, in her book *Overtreated: Why Too Much Medicine Is Making Us Sicker and Poorer*[116] makes a convincing and provocative case for why the USA is suffering the adverse effects of too much health care. With detailed examples on the excessive overuse of screening programs, diagnostic services, drugs, surgery, and all the hospital care that these entail, she makes a solid case for why health care, like any medication, needs to be taken in its proper dose.

However, all is not so bleak. The report notes that the US does not need more high-tech solutions, but smarter ways to deliver health care. It notes that one key to saving the US healthcare system could be a widespread adoption of "tools that deliver reliable clinical knowledge to patients." In other words, if all healthcare consumers, including physicians, nurses and other clinicians, and healthcare organizations and administrators better under-stood the effectiveness, safety, and comparative value of what they were buying, then they could be vastly wiser consumers of health care.

They could be more effective purchasers of that health care, too. According to the Institute of Medicine (IOM), a non-profit US organization that "asks and answers the nation's most pressing questions about health and health care,"[117] if clinicians adhered to evidence-based practices, they'd trim as much as 30 per cent from the nation's healthcare bill. Additionally, if "evidence was consist-ently applied to treatment recommendations and patient manage-ment," not only would the nation as a whole save money, but there would probably be an improvement in the overall health of the population, rich and poor.[118]

The authors of the *Best Care at Lower Cost* report make this important point: "America's healthcare system has become far too complex and costly to continue business as usual."[119] Consumers and clinicians need knowledge to be aware of their options and to make the best decisions. Among other prescriptions, the authors stress the use of what they call "decision-support tools and know-ledge management systems at point of care."

That sounds like a mission for the Cochrane Collaboration.

A Fantastic Digestive System

WHILE I'M talking here about the US health system, the princi-ples could apply to any national healthcare system that has to deal with maximizing the effect of its healthcare spending and doing so in an affordable and sustainable way for its entire population. The USA is an outlier in many aspects of its healthcare system, but one of the more obvious and egregious aspects of US health care is the size of its pharmaceutical expenditures. The USA has the highest per capita drug costs on the planet – head and shoul-ders above the next country (Canada).

American drug companies are politically active, and the drug industry has a well-funded lobby machine that finances clinical and drug research, Key Opinion Leaders (known by the acronym KOLs), and disease and patient groups. American consumers experience a daily onslaught of direct-to-consumer advertising of drugs. Hospitals have massive marketing budgets to compete for patients, and the patients they attract are seen as "cost centers."

Andrew Herxheimer has seen firsthand how poorly physicians perform in prescribing. He knows how skewed physicians' perceptions of drugs can be – of both the beneficial and the harmful effects. This issue has been on his RADAR for more than half a century.[120]

Herxheimer qualified as a physician in England in 1949, and worked for a short while in the US health system in Utah, USA. He remembers when the *Medical Letter on Drugs and Therapeutics* (first published in 1959) began.

He said, "It had been going a year or two, and I thought, 'That's important. Every country needs that.'" Determined to start one like it in the UK, he was adamant that he "didn't want a medical publisher to do it because medical publishers depend on industry. I wanted an industry-independent publisher." So what did he do? He said, "I asked the Consumers Association, which was then quite young, and to my surprise and gratification, they did it." He went on to create and act as chief editor for the *Drug and Therapeutics Bulletin*, starting about 1962.

Herxheimer found that his independent bulletin became an important vehicle for getting impartial drug information to physicians. He used it as a vehicle to get the WHO onboard, as well.

As he saw it, as the world's premier health policymaking organization, the WHO needed to be proactive and engaged in actively advising nations on the value of independent drug information and on how to set up bulletins; also to provide information for professionals. Amid this, Herxheimer has never lost sight of the ultimate purpose of all this: to inform medical care that bene-fits all of us, we 'consumers' of health care.

Herxheimer has been a prominent member of Health Action International (HAI) since its inception in 1981. HAI is probably the strongest global voice on access to medicines and high-quality medicine information. A former employee of HAI and long-time colleague of his is epidemiologist Barbara Mintzes who works at the University of Sydney, in Australia.[121] She has a unique per-spective on Andrew Herxheimer.

She told me why he differs from others who develop and support drug information initiatives: "Often when people reach prominence in their field, they get distracted by all the trappings, and even if they started out with a commitment to social change, it doesn't necessarily stick. With Andrew, it always has. He's al-ways had a dual commitment to the science and to consumer and patient rights."

This commitment is probably most evident in his involvement in creating DIPEx, a group that encourages patients to share their health experiences. He's also a co-convenor of Cochrane's Adverse Events Methods Group, the role of which is to help ad-vance ways of finding and communicating the adverse effects of health treatments. Since those treatments – often drugs – always involve both a prescriber and a consumer, he maintains that "the Cochrane Collaboration has to find out what is actually best for the people – for the final users and the intermediate users, the professionals."

He is keenly aware of the incredible accumulation of health-care knowledge over the last 60 years, which is still growing at an enormous rate and threatens to overwhelm us all. The problem, he says, is that it's "undigested," adding with a glint in his eye, "The Cochrane Collaboration is the best digestive system for all the knowledge that we have."

Finding Out What's Effective First

Staying on the topic of digestive systems, it's time to meet a gastroenterologist whose work focuses on digestive systems and their disorders. He has also been frustrated at times with a lack of available information, and knows how crucial reliable evidence can be in making healthcare decisions.

Ronald Koretz is saddened by what he has seen happen to medicine in his lifetime. The retired gastroenterologist worked for 32 years at the Olive View-UCLA Medical Center in Sylmar, California. He's old enough to remember when doctors made house calls.

He's particularly disturbed by what he sees as the preoccupation of physicians these days. "They seem to be focused on making money," he says, adding, "For many doctors, income is more important than outcome, and that bothers me."

While Koretz does not preach state-sponsored health care, he spent his career in public hospitals that treated people who had no health insurance. "I really enjoyed the idea that I was doing my bit to help my fellow man."

He remembers reading a short blurb in 1994 in the *Annals of Internal Medicine* about this new thing called the Cochrane Collaboration. The blurb raised a question that caught his fancy: "How would you like to be involved in an organization where you do a lot of work but you get no credit?"

"You know," he laughs, "that's my kind of organization. The idea that the whole is greater than any sum of the parts. So I called them and said, 'What do you guys *do*?' I had no idea what these guys were all about."

Whoever he talked to didn't clarify things. "I had no clue what they were talking about." So the woman he spoke to invited him to "just come up to Hamilton [a Canadian city about 70 kilometres southwest of Toronto, where the Collaboration was having its annual Colloquium]. Come to the Colloquium and see what it's like." That seemed reasonable, so he went – and quickly found that he was in his element.

Koretz had had plenty of experience with how challenging it could be to find quality information on various interventions. In particular, he'd been searching out information on the benefits of total parenteral nutrition (TPN) – the intravenous administration of artificial nutrition – but had found only a limited number of randomized controlled trials (RCTs) on the topic.

The RCT evidence – mostly small or methodologically imperfect trials – did not show that TPN had any effect on patients at all. He admits that, at the time, "I didn't really know anything about evidence-based medicine. I knew that randomized trials were different and better, but that's all I knew."

One theme repeats in the stories of the people in the Cochrane Collaboration: they decide that they want to know everything about a particular medical niche. After a lot of hard work, largely done in obscurity, digging through studies, contacting researchers, and learning everything possible about the research on a topic, they become the world's acknowledged experts on the topic.

Koretz admitted that this obsession with finding good evidence in the medical literature made him a natural "bosom buddy" to Iain Chalmers. He said, "We had the same concept that the healthcare system was getting out of control," and added, "The best way to handle it was to use the evidence to decide where we would or wouldn't spend money."

Now retired and in his early 70s, Koretz stays involved as one of Cochrane's principal reviewers with the Hepato-Biliary Group (a group focused on liver and biliary diseases). He expresses no vanity when he admits that he's probably one of their more rigorous review editors. "When the reviews come out," he says, "I go through every comma and period. But mostly I ask, 'Does this make sense?'"

Every Secret Has a Reason

As to why the work of the Cochrane Collaboration hasn't really taken off in the USA as it has in other countries, Koretz says that the reviews produced by Cochrane might be seen as a "threat to the healthcare system in the US." Our conversation turns to doctors and he explains that maybe "the reason they don't want to use [Cochrane reviews] is that they would have to admit they shouldn't do what they are doing."

For example, he talks about one of the Cochrane reviews he worked on concerning the use of interferon treatment for people with hepatitis C. The review showed that interferon did not result in improved morbidity (developing liver failure or needing a liver transplant) or decreased mortality caused by liver disease. The one thing the trials do show is that the treatment can lead to clearance of the virus in a small minority of patients.[122]

Then he told me that when they looked closer at just the higher-quality studies – those deemed to have a low risk of bias – there was a surprise: more people treated with interferon died. "The treatment did not help, and the surrogate outcome (disappearance of the virus from the blood stream) failed validation." This was an expensive, heavily used treatment strongly favored by many of Koretz's colleagues who treated hepatitis C patients.

Koretz admits that many of his colleagues and patients worked under a false assumption: if you get hepatitis C, you're dead. "Actually the vast majority of patients won't get into trouble," he said, adding that often patients are not told that.

He emphasizes that, sometimes, the truth emerging from a systematic review is hard to swallow. Because he feels that Cochrane reviews are rigorously done to the highest of standards, they'll often find that their conclusions are at odds with what people think. In Koretz's words, the reviews will often "say a particular treatment doesn't work, or that we have no evidence that it works."

He feels disappointed that many medical professionals disregard the results of high-quality systematic reviews. "It's surprising to me that an organization with the intellectual power of Cochrane is so disregarded." He says, "If you go to meetings and talk about a Cochrane review, they'll accept it is a Cochrane review, but then they'll go home and do whatever they want."

Looking forward, Koretz echoes what others have said. "Maybe in ten years, Cochrane will be a huge player here [in the USA], but it remains somewhat sidelined at the moment."

As of 2013, there were only small pots of funding to support Cochrane activities in the USA. The US Cochrane Centers would like to see more funding, specifically for infrastructure support, as well as for helping to expand Cochrane research in the USA beyond existing review groups already working in HIV/AIDS and neonatal medicine.

In the USA, Koretz's home country, there are demands for spending in many new areas of health care – for new drugs, new surgical techniques, and so on. There is also a growing push to ask: How about finding out what is effective first?

The Investment of a Lifetime?

Why should governments want to invest in the Cochrane Collaboration? A good answer to that question comes from someone who considers investing in the Collaboration a good idea.

Andy Haines is a professor of public health and primary care at the London School of Hygiene and Tropical Medicine in England.[123] In the early 1990s, Haines was on secondment, acting as the director of research and development at the NHS Executive, North Thames. He says, "I was approached at the time by Iain Chalmers about the possibility of funding for, in those days, the Cochrane Centre. I was very enthusiastic about the whole concept and could see immediately from the point of view of being a researcher, but then also a research funder, how crucial it was to synthesize in a rigorous way research evidence."

He adds, "There have been far too many kinds of false leads given by individual studies, often giving us very biased views of research. So I was very convinced very early on this is an important way to go."

Any regrets? I wondered. Haines, also known as Professor Sir Andrew Haines, doesn't hesitate. "I think it was probably the best investment I ever made in my career as a research funder." He says that the "30,000 pounds or something" that the NHS initially invested in the Collaboration has made an "extraordinary contribution" to global health.

Haines and Chalmers are on the same page when it comes to the priority of systematic reviews. He said: "I've always tried to support the importance of systematic reviews as a sort of absolutely essential first step before you embark on new research."

Things are not always so systematic at the highest levels of health policy making, such as the World Health Organization. Says Haines: "There had been rather an *ad hoc* approach to many recommendations and guidelines coming out of WHO." The WHO puts out recommendations for countries around the world to follow, helping poorer countries who might not have the bench strength or resources to systematically review evidence. "In the old days, perhaps ten years… ago, people would convene a group of experts and then they would come up with some sort of recommendations, and so that obviously had to change." It was obvious because, as we have seen many times, a group of experts can be very wrong. If they aren't thoroughly grounding their recommendations in systematic evidence, that could harm people.

Haines says that, since then, the "whole culture has changed quite dramatically in WHO, and now there is much stronger emphasis on rigor and transparent guidelines based on systematic reviews" – a culture to which, he says, "the Cochrane Collaboration is absolutely central."

Reasons for Hope

I demonstrated to my kids what the word *alliteration* meant when I told them that I was going to a meeting in the USA in October, 2010. The name of the meeting (I wasn't making this up) was the "Campbell and Cochrane Collaboration Colloquium in Keystone, Colorado." I was on a roll, so I continued: why not attend a cool yet collegial conference with keeners coming from all corners of the Cochrane and Campbell communities? Ok, Dad. We get it.

But you probably couldn't have found a more picturesque and challenging setting for a meeting. One of the organizers of that conference was Bob Dellavalle, a dermatologist in Denver, Colorado, who at that time had been doing reviews with Cochrane for about ten years.[124]

Dellavalle said that Keystone was a unique meeting because it was jointly organized with the Campbell Collaboration. Campbell is a sister organization to Cochrane and carries out systematic reviews of evidence in the behavioral world, similar to what the Cochrane Collaboration does in health care. This Colloquium in Colorado was the first time the two organizations shared a major conference.

The history of the Campbell Collaboration probably warrants a separate book of its own. One of its creators is Bob Boruch, a professor at the University of Pennsylvania. An early and influential proponent of using randomized trials to assess educational and social programs, he met Iain Chalmers at Cochrane's first US Colloquium, in Baltimore, in 1998[125].

Chalmers knew of Boruch's work and asked him if he'd consider starting a sister organization to prepare and maintain systematic reviews of social and behavioral interventions. Chalmers suggested that this new organization should be named after

Donald Campbell (1916–96), a Northwestern University psychologist under whom Boruch had studied.

Donald T. Campbell was an appropriate inspiration for this group, and, like Archie Cochrane, a strong advocate for an experimental approach to almost everything. Campbell describes a near-utopian, "non-dogmatic" world in a famous essay, "The Experimenting Society," which like Archie Cochrane's *Effectiveness and Efficiency*, sets out a rationale for humans developing what he calls an "accountable, challengeable and due-process society."[126]

Bob Boruch said that a "game changer" example of a Campbell Collaboration systematic review relates to certain popular programs in the USA that try to prevent kids from choosing a life of crime or drugs.[127] Such programs work by scaring the delinquency out of kids through prison tours led by hardened criminals who have lots of tattoos and scary stories of life inside the slammer. At least that's the reasoning behind programs like *Scared Straight!* that are supposed to do what the name suggests. Boruch said that *Scared Straight!*-type programs are "very popular with schools, cops, moms and dads."

The problem was, once the program got a good going-over by Anthony Petrosino and his Campbell Collaboration colleagues, who did a meta-analysis of nine RCTs of *Scared Straight!*-type programs, the evidence indicated the exact opposite.[128] Basically, scaring the bejeesus out of kids headed for delinquency makes things worse. In fact, the programs make it more likely that kids end up in trouble. *Scared Curious* might be a more appropriate title.

There is a lot of common ground between the Cochrane and Campbell Collaborations, both premised on the idea that when you actually collect and meta-analyze good quality research, you find surprises – such as pretty good proof that you're hurting the very people you're hoping to help. And like the Cochrane Collaboration, the folks at Campbell are major proponents of high-quality evaluations. They push governments to invest in proper RCTs of interventions, which can deliver the real goods on whether a program works or not.

The Keystone Colloquium in 2010 provided a unique opportunity to get the two groups together. Bob Dellavalle said that the conference helped both organizations to discover "how they relate and how they are different."

Dellavalle was by all accounts an exceptional organizer and pulled off this joint conference with barely a hitch. When I asked him what that was like he said, "I learned a lot about how to bring 800 people from around the world to high altitude where they might get altitude sickness. And how to have a good time in the natural scenery of the mountains."

His area of research is skin disease, and his interest in systematic evidence arose when he wanted to look at medications to prevent melanoma. He credits Hywel Williams, the founding co-ordinating editor of the Cochrane Skin Group, based in Nottingham, England, for giving him the training and the inspiration he needed to help on a Cochrane systematic review. He said that the Cochrane approach was the "right thing to do" and he calls himself a "true believer" in the mission of the organization.

Dellavalle emphasizes that the biggest effect of the Cochrane Collaboration in his mind is that "it continues to be the gold standard for systematic reviews." Having reliable and trustworthy evidence is important because "we have fewer resources to devote to our medical services worldwide." The problem in the USA, and in every other nation in the world, is to balance the appropriate use of resources for health care, and that's why gold-standard evidence is so important.

He sees a huge advantage in the advent of electronic literature searches, where, he says, he and his colleagues can look at the world's evidence and avoid basing their medical care on "customs passed down from one physician to the next physician generation."

Just before the Keystone Colloquium opened, Dellavalle and the editor in chief of the *Cochrane Library*, David Tovey, published a commentary setting out how an expanded Cochrane Collaboration could help serve the healthcare information needs of the United States.[129]

They wrote, "The Cochrane Colloquium's return to the USA provides cause of celebration and reflection," and, like many of those who have had leadership positions in the Collaboration, they were eager for more ways for the Collaboration to engage in the USA. American contributors have been an essential part of the Collaboration from the very beginning, including people such as Kay Dickersin, Tom Chalmers, Roger Soll, Andy Oxman (long transplanted to Norway), Lisa Bero, and others.

The US taxpayer has been involved since the Cochrane Collaboration's start, in 1993, with money from the National Institutes of Health (NIH) helping to fund various review groups and fields. The NIH also helped with the first ten years of the *Cochrane Central Register of Controlled Trials*. According to Kay Dickersin, the NIH is not a small player, and over the years "has supported Cochrane entities to the tune of tens of millions of dollars."

Of course, there remains a vast and growing amount of world medical literature to be examined and put into systematic reviews. Some people say that this could be accomplished if all of the NIH institutes were onboard with supporting Cochrane reviews. The one big thing that remains on the wish list for Cochrane operations in the USA is infrastructure support: the day-to-day administration, educational, and managerial work that requires paid staff, designated offices, and stable, predictable funding.

Since NIH is organized by institutes and not across health

areas generally, it's hard for any single NIH institute to agree to cover infrastructure. In contrast to other countries, such as Canada, Brazil or the UK, where government funders have found ways to pay for the infrastructure for Cochrane centres and methods groups, this remains an unfulfilled dream in the USA.

Another major item on the US Cochrane wish list is to have the *Cochrane Library* made available for free to all who live there. If you're a citizen in the UK, India or Australia, you get free access to the full *Cochrane Library*. If you're a citizen of the USA? Sorry. Unless you live in Wyoming. Unbelievably, Wyoming is the only US state with a site licence to the *Cochrane Library* and Cochrane reviews are freely available to all Wyoming citizens.

Canada currently doesn't pay for access to a national site license to the *Cochrane Library, though there are site licences for Nova Scotia and New Brunswick.* Even though Jeremy Grimshaw, who possibly wears more hats than nearly anyone in the Collaboration (at the time of writing he was the co-chair of the Steering Group, director of the Canadian Cochrane Centre, and coordinating editor of the Effective Practice and Organisation of Care Group), has been instrumental in securing critical Canadian government investment in the Collaboration, he hasn't yet convinced Ottawa that a national site license is the way to go. As this book goes to print, the funding for Cochrane Canada, supplied by the Canadian Institutes of Health Research, has been halted, though talks are continuing to see what ongoing support might look like.

Various countries' leaderships tend to be partial to home-grown solutions. In the USA, some agencies that fund health services research (such as the well-known Agency for Healthcare Research and Quality, or AHRQ) also direct their own evidence synthesis programs, similar to the Collaboration. Canada has CADTH – the Canadian Agency for Drugs and Technologies in Health, which also does evidence synthesis for government.

In 1997, the AHRQ created evidence based practice centres – and for this reason (among others), it has not yet supported US-based Cochrane groups, beyond awarding several conference grants. Hardly the infrastructure support needed.

Since the Collaboration's beginning, there have been four US Cochrane Centers – in Baltimore, San Francisco, San Antonio and New England. Only two survive, and they are both hanging by a thread because of lack of government funding. In 2012, eight Cochrane entities were registered in the USA, including review groups specializing in benign prostatic disease and urologic cancers, eyes and vision, HIV/AIDS, and neonatal research. There is also a field focusing on complementary and alternative medicine. About 1,500 US-based review authors were contributing to the *Cochrane Library*, and almost 70 per cent of Cochrane review groups had at least one US-based editor.

David Tovey and Bob Dellavalle remind us that Cochrane reviews in the USA have had a substantial effect: "The USA represents the largest number of users of the *Cochrane Library* (in 2009, over 1.8 million visits, constituting 33% of the whole), while top-10 US medical schools and 40 of the top 50 have licence to the *Cochrane Library*."[130]

Kay Dickersin, who has probably done more to seek funding for Cochrane operations in the USA than anyone, thinks that if the AHRQ and other funders contribute much, much more, then Cochrane contributors in the USA could produce much, much more.

There might yet be reason for hope. President Obama's *Affordable Care Act* portends significant healthcare reform, including a substantial dedication of resources for comparative effectiveness research, as well as research on the needs and demands of patients.

The Patient-Centered Outcomes Research Institute (PCORI, found at pcori.org), as its name implies, is a hopeful new non-profit funding agency with a mission to involve patients and clinicians. The goal is to produce research that is meaningful for these end-users – in other words, all of us. PCORI is premised on the idea that medical and health research has often drifted too far away from what is meaningful and valuable to the patients, and that without a concerted effort to focus on what people actually want, genuine healthcare reform may never happen.

The other US innovation, which has been driven by the US Cochrane Center, is the group Consumers United for Evidence-based Healthcare (us.cochrane.org/CUE), which seeks to stimulate thoughtful participation from grassroots consumers. Its goal is to get consumers working with and understanding the Cochrane Collaboration's product: systematic evidence. It is really about producing powerful advocates for effective, safe, and cost-effective health care – which is often at odds with what is promoted by consumer organizations that depend on support from the pharmaceutical or the health-insurance industries.

It seems a hopeful time to be involved in healthcare research in the USA. Many people, like Kay Dickersin, are optimistic that these innovations will do what many past reforms haven't done: stem the waste, duplication, and excess in US health care. When you remember that as much as US $2 billion daily is wasted on unnecessary, unneeded, and perhaps unwanted health care, these reforms cannot come soon enough.

The USA likes to be known as a country of innovation. But when it comes to health care, what kind of innovation do US citizens most need? British physician and medical pundit Ben Goldacre might have put it best when he wrote that "the notion of systematic review – looking at the totality of evidence – is quietly one of the most important innovations in medicine over the past 30 years."[131]

Can the Cochrane Collaboration become more prominent

in the USA, pushing for more support for, and use of, the systematic reviews that have defined it? Is it too grandiose a dream to hope that the USA as a nation will live up to the Keystone Colloquium's motto and "bring evidence-based decision-making to new heights?"

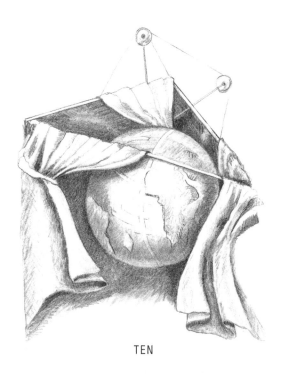

TEN

Global Perspectives:
The Need for Relevant Information

*"What made medicine fool people for so long was
that its successes were prominently displayed and
its mistakes (literally) buried."*

— Nassim Nicholas Taleb

PAUL GARNER is a professor at the Liverpool School of Tropical Medicine in the UK and the co-ordinating editor of Cochrane's Infectious Diseases Group. He may also be the only Cochranite whose connection to the Collaboration goes back to the day he was born.[132]

After Garner was born, his mother kept in touch with the

midwives who had helped at his delivery. One of them, Ann Stewart, knew Iain Chalmers mainly through her role in midwifery in the UK, where she'd worked in the 1990s as the most senior midwifery officer in the English National Board of Nursing, Midwifery and Health Visiting. When Stewart found out that young Garner was working on studying the issue of birthweight in Papua New Guinea, she called Chalmers and told him that he should get to know "one of her babies."

Garner said, "So I got an overseas phone call in my office in Madang from a man I didn't know, asking me what I was doing. He wanted to know about malaria and whether I might want to look at whether preventing malaria helps improve the health of newborns."

Garner was intrigued and he told me that he started going to Oxford and meeting with Iain Chalmers while he was writing his thesis. "Iain kept talking about doing a systematic review and going to the library and searching the library by hand for trials in this area. I had no idea what he was driving at."

But soon the light came on for him. He said that one day he sat down with Chalmers, and together they assembled the data from six or seven trials systematically into a table. Suddenly, "I could see the whole point of what he was trying to do. It was very important to me at that time," and was something that left him absolutely "hooked."

Later, he remembers reading an editorial in the *British Medical Journal* (*BMJ*) calling for people to collaborate with this new international group being formed. "I was sitting in a hotel room in Lahore [Pakistan] reading the *BMJ* editorial announcing the setting up of the Cochrane Centre in Oxford. I had just bought a portable printer for work overseas, and the first letter I wrote was to Iain saying that I wanted to help, and that it was very important that it included health problems from developing countries and people from developing countries in the process. These are slightly different, but both are often forgotten when new initiatives are at a planning stage."

His group, the Cochrane Infectious Diseases Group, which focuses on research on tropical diseases endemic to developing countries, was one of the first to register with the Collaboration, in May, 1994. He points to this to demonstrate that the Collaboration has had a longstanding interest in and "commitment to problems of illness which have the greatest burden." This focus reflected Chalmers' own philosophy and commitment throughout his career, dating from his work in refugee camps in Gaza, Palestine.

Stop Competing and Start Working Together

The inaugural meeting of the Collaboration, chaired by Peter Tugwell, made an explicit commitment that the organization would seek wider engagement and engage developing countries. Garner felt that the meeting had been inspiring because there were so many enthusiastic people from "all over the place," and he recalled that he found it both "energizing and powerful." His eyes shine with enthusiasm when he adds, "It was a privilege to be there, really, and you felt as if you were at the beginning of something that was pretty exciting."

From his perspective of working in academia, Garner has a deep understanding of competition. In academic settings, there is often intense competition for grants, for positions, for prestige, and for power. In fact, some say that universities can be among the most political and competitive places in our societies. He said, "The concept of collaborating was a radical concept in academia at the time. I remember sitting down with Iain and the heads of the two departments in an institution which I worked in, to try and get them working together on this issue. After the meeting was over, one of the departmental heads came up to me and said, 'Paul, I would perhaps be careful about sharing this with the other departments, because they may nick this idea.'" Garner shook his head. "This is how academic institutions are."

"The spirit of collaboration [in Cochrane] was refreshing. The ideas were also anti-authoritarian and anti-expert." He grinned when he recalled, "Iain was described in Sunday newspapers as being the leader of an obstetric Baader Meinhof gang [a German leftist guerrilla group]. And so, for young people coming into the field of medical research, it was refreshing to know that the worst rebels there had something important to say; that we could communicate with and identify with very strongly."

Cholera, Malaria, and
What Systematic Reviews Can Tell Us

Dehydration is a big killer in the developing world. Children with cholera or other diarrheal diseases lose too much body fluid to diarrhea and die. In 1971, civil war in what is now Bangladesh forced more than 350,000 people into refugee camps. The medical teams were inundated. It was impossible to provide intravenous fluids to all of the 3,000 people suffering from cholera. Dr. Dilip Mahalanabis had the foresight to ask his staff to distribute oral rehydration solution (ORS) instead and direct mothers to give their children as much fluid as they could take. The death rate plummeted quickly.

ORS is a formula of sugar and salts to be mixed with clean water. It comes in a packet. Because delivery of ORS does not require medical staff, its use is appropriate in an emergency situation. So successful has ORS been that diarrhea as a cause of infant death has dropped to second place worldwide (behind pneumonia). Despite this success, for a long time the question of what exactly should be put in ORS remained unanswered. What was the optimal solution?

Paul Garner recalled, "A number of trials... testing a formula that had less salt in it had been done, but people were still arguing whether or not to change the formula. Obviously the question was being asked because that's why people were doing the trials, but the results were mixed, and the World Health Organization weren't sure what to do and they asked us to carry out a Cochrane review. The meta-analysis we did helped show very clearly that the newer, slightly less salty solution was better than the formula that was currently being used."

As a direct result of this analysis, the formula for rehydration-salt solution changed globally. "We showed clearly there was a consistency between the trials. Fewer children needed IV infusion, and fewer vomited with the new formula. This tweaking of an important intervention improves the treatment of a major cause of death in developing countries; so it's contributing to decreasing mortality in these groups."

Paul Garner clearly enjoys what he's doing, and he likes the impact his work can have in the area of infectious diseases. "The effects you're dealing with are often quite large, so it's quite a satisfying area to work in," he told me.

It has been, however, a struggle, especially in an uphill battle with the specialists, Garner explains. This results in tropical medicine still lagging behind mainstream medicine in accepting the value of independent, carefully done systematic reviews. Garner recalls, "When we started doing this, people said, 'You cannot do it. It's a waste of time. Malaria is so varied. You cannot do systematic reviews.' But the people that said this were the people that were doing trials. This does not make sense. If they didn't want generalized lessons out of it, why do the trials? So we've challenged them over the years and have clearly demonstrated impacts of well-done, systematic reviews. They are now part of the picture." He adds, "The systematic reviews won't tell you everything that you need to know in order to make decisions, but they tell you an awful lot."

TB and DOT: What the Evidence Says

With a bright smile and a steady gaze, Jimmy Volmink tells me how he came to be the director of the South African Cochrane Centre, based in Cape Town, South Africa.[133]

"It was 1993. The first time I came into contact with Iain Chalmers was also when I heard about the Collaboration. It was an accident that happened in Oxford. I had arrived in Oxford on a research fellowship with my family. It was around about August–September of that year, and I was cycling very slowly down one of the roads called Middle Way."

Middle Way is a relatively short and narrow street in Oxford that lies between two larger thoroughfares, Woodstock Road and Banbury Road – hence its name. It's also the street on which sits the Summertown Pavilion, the headquarters of the UK Cochrane Centre and (until March 2015, when it relocated to London) the international Cochrane Operations Unit.

Volmink: "A gentleman came walking in the opposite direction. Even before he got to me, he greeted me very enthusiastically, and then we struck up a conversation, which I quite enjoyed. We spoke about all sorts of things, and he ended up welcoming me to Oxford, pointed out where he worked, and said that he'd like to tell me something about what he does there. Would I visit sometime in the future?"

Volmink shakes his head a bit and smiles: "I reflected on this and thought, 'Well, here's an Englishman who speaks to strangers. That's kind of odd.' And he didn't look like he was crazy or anything. And, in fact, quite the opposite. He seemed a very kind and intelligent sort of person, and I was quite intrigued by this encounter. Two weeks later, I went to visit him at his office. He turned out to be Iain Chalmers. Within five minutes, I think he convinced me [that] for the rest of my life, I'd want to do Cochrane reviews. And that's how I got to know about Cochrane."

This all transpired a few months after the inaugural Cochrane meeting in 1993. Volmink said he'd "vaguely heard about the Collaboration, but I didn't connect the two when I met this gentleman." He said that once Iain Chalmers explained to him what Cochrane was all about, "it just seemed such an exciting, ambitious project, and so highly sensible that I thought, you know, why didn't I think of this earlier?"

Volmink was excited and eager to contribute, especially because it was made very clear at the start that this initiative wasn't going to be focused exclusively on the concerns of the rich developed world, and that, to be successful, the Collaboration required global participation.

He was probably thinking of the burden of tuberculosis (TB) in his part of the world. After all, TB is most associated with and most confined to pockets of poverty. It is rare in the developed world, but common in developing countries.

TB has been with humankind for millennia. The disease known historically as "consumption" was a widespread cause of death in the nineteenth century. An active TB infection can cause a chronic cough, fever and night sweats, as well as weight loss (hence the consumption). Even in the modern era, with effective drugs and preventive therapies, TB still kills millions every year.

Volmink admits that his first Cochrane review, published in 1997, was quite controversial at the time. It was a review of something called Directly Observed Therapy (DOT). The biggest problem in treating TB is ensuring that the patient takes a full course of treatment, which might involve taking a pill every day for six to nine months. In some countries, people stop treatment prematurely, which gives their TB a chance to rebound.

Even worse, the patient can develop multiple drug-resistant forms of TB that can be extremely difficult or even impossible to treat. The rationale behind DOT was that, if someone were there to actually observe patients taking their daily pill, the treatment would be much more consistent and effective.

From Jimmy Volmink's perspective, the WHO "strongly promoted this [DOT] approach. They said people couldn't be trusted to take the medication by themselves and needed to be watched while they took their medication... I thought, 'Well, I wonder what the evidence is for that.'" He discussed this with Paul Garner, and together the two decided to carry out a Cochrane review of DOT for TB.

The reason why this review was considered controversial was, as Volmink said, "primarily because we discovered there was no good evidence to support that intervention." When they published this fact in 1997, he said, "The WHO and others were extremely upset about that, because they felt that the review undermined their position on this. What was interesting was that a lot of people did send us e-mails and letters of appreciation because they had also felt this was a strange kind of way to approach care for people with tuberculosis." At that time, directly observing treatment was not an approach used for patients suffering from other diseases.

Volmink said, "The WHO was sold on it [the DOT approach] because it seemed to be a safe way to treat people whom they regarded to be a great public health risk, and they wanted to ensure that they could see people taking the medication. But it turns out," he continues, "that, in fact, that's probably not true; that you may be driving away some people by adopting that sort of policy."

As Volmink explains it, when you look at the research that focused on what's called "adherence to therapy" (an area that was a strong theme of Dave Sackett's research early in his career), you find that most of the research isn't of high enough quality to determine if adherence is actually effective. The world lacks good, definitive research results pointing to patients' adherence to therapy as certain to save lives.

He says, "When we did the review, we said, 'Well, let's look at all interventions out there that are intended to promote adherence to therapy for people with tuberculosis. So we didn't just look at DOT. And we looked at trials of other types of interventions ranging from education to packaging of medication and a few other things, and in total found about 10 or 11 trials that had tested interventions, but there wasn't a single one that looked at DOT in that sort of rigorous way."

He adds, "The only available evidence was really largely observational uncontrolled studies and hunches really that people had that this might have been a good thing in the past because some people had introduced it, and they saw adherence rates going up, and they felt that was due to the observation."

Observational studies can have their merit as well, but are obviously not as strong as a randomized trial where biases of both the researcher and the patient can be controlled. After this first review, Jimmy and his team carried out another, looking specifically at the observational research; looking very carefully at the observational studies in which DOT had been introduced. They found that the DOT program had been studied "alongside a number of other interventions, including massive increases in funding of TB programs, celebrations of people who have completed therapy, and the like – so a number of co-interventions – and it was impossible to say which of these was, in fact, responsible for the changes that we were seeing."

I wondered whether that was worth all the trouble. Wasn't it most vital to get the medication to people whose lives could be saved, regardless of how the distribution programs work? The fact is, TB does have a long history of high-quality research programs. It is such a deadly disease and has affected millions. Volmink reminded me, "When Archie Cochrane initially handed out awards for the most evidence-based and the least evidence-based specialties, the TB specialists were singled out for an award for being the most evidence-based."

Events subsequent to the publication of the DOT review appear still to be somewhat award-worthy, à la Archie Cochrane. Volmink goes on to say that, since the review's first publication, a number of trials have been carried out to determine whether or not DOT is an effective treatment protocol. The current version of the review includes 11 randomized controlled trials of DOT and taken together, they still provide no evidence to support a DOT-based treatment policy.

So what is it about work in TB that promotes such an evidence-based approach? Volmink's theory: "They had conducted a number of trials, showing that various drugs and drug combinations were effective, and they could base their treatments and strategy regimes on very good evidence. The trouble with TB is that the adherence has always been a problem." Getting people to take the medication has always been one of the greatest challenges. There are other challenges, too. Trying accurately and simply to diagnose people quickly is a problem. Also, both new diagnostic methods and better drugs are urgently needed.

Volmink says, "Within the last few years, we've seen a much greater emphasis on trying to find new ways of diagnosing TB, because the methods that have been used are very old – 50 years old or more, and also the drugs are very old. There haven't been new drugs for TB for a very long time."

Sadly, the war on TB seems a losing battle. There has been very little decrease in the incidence of the disease. The situation is complicated by the HIV epidemic: HIV infection is considered "one of the drivers of tuberculosis because it [TB] is an opportunistic infection which is influenced by the presence of an immune problem compromising the immune system," says Volmink.

Solving this problem is not made easier by pockets of dire

poverty in the world. Problems of overcrowding and poor nutrition have made tuberculosis particularly hard to fight.

I wonder why Volmink doesn't lose hope against such a formidable foe as TB. He tells me, "I realize that TB in one way is not unique. There have been many other diseases that have taken a very long time for people to find a really important cure and a lasting solution for."

He sees a parallel in the long time it has taken for healthcare professionals to apply effective therapies. He reminds me of scurvy, a disease that was devastating to sailors centuries ago. Volmink finds it encouraging that even when "very good evidence was produced that oranges and lemons cure scurvy and can prevent scurvy, it took more than 100 years for that evidence to be adopted into practice and for people to routinely receive the therapy. So, sometimes things take a long time, but people have to press on and believe that you will eventually win the battle."

When Volmink first became involved in the Collaboration, he didn't feel encouraged by the fact that the newly-created database of systematic reviews contained "very little... that had any relevance to Africa, or to other developing countries, for that matter." When he left Oxford to go back to South Africa, he already had a plan to establish the South African Cochrane Centre, resolving that "we would prioritize the conditions of importance to Africa." He recognized that he had a lot of help, particularly working with other Cochrane review groups, especially the Infectious Diseases Group, as well as the HIV/AIDS Group.

Over the years, he said, they have "been able to substantially increase the number of reviews that are relevant to Africa in areas such as HIV, tuberculosis, malaria, some health systems issues that we've looked at, and nutritional issues." There has been a lot of progress and the *Cochrane Library* does contain good information to inform decisions and management of problems in Africa, but there is still a problem of the low number and quality of reviews on relevant topics.

Volmink urges more engagement and says that "very few [review authors] come from Africa where the problem is, and so the question is: how relevant is this evidence to the local situation? And that's a challenge that we frequently face."

About Cochrane Volmink says, "One of the things that attracted me to Cochrane was not only the mission. It had a clear mission, and that's great; it's very idealistic and very ambitious and all of that's very exciting – but also very exciting is the nature of the people that are involved in Cochrane. I have found them to be some of the most inspiring people that I've ever met. I think they are people who are enormously generous in terms of sharing their knowledge and skills."

I asked Volmink about the Colloquium in Cape Town. "Yeah, that was the first and last Colloquium I organized. And it was, first of all, a tremendous privilege to do that, but it was also terrifying. I've never organized any conference or been the main person responsible for a conference before, and before I left Oxford (which was at the end of 1996) Iain Chalmers had said to me, 'Well, I think you should organize the 2000 Colloquium,' and I thought he was joking, because we were just about to start the Cochrane Centre in South Africa in 1997 when I got back. And so, almost from day one... we had to think about organizing this conference."

Was it worth it, I wondered. Volmink: "I think it was a tremendously positive experience to host this with people from Cochrane from all over the world coming and joining us. It was a great opportunity for us to draw in people from South Africa and other African countries; to get them to meet people involved in Cochrane, and I think that had a lasting impact on many people in South Africa who have since become involved with Cochrane."

He says the Cape Town Colloquium is to thank for getting

more attention from the Medical Research Council of South Africa which funds the South African Cochrane Centre. Volmink: "I think it was the Colloquium that made a huge impression on them. Just meeting the people, understanding the high quality of the individuals involved; the fact that they were really leaders in the field of evidence-based medicine and clinical epidemiology of the world, and the value of the product that we produce... I think all of those things could be showcased, and people could understand it much better because they were there. They could experience it firsthand. So it was great."

Much has been accomplished by Volmink and others he has brought into the fold since 1993. Even more has yet to be accomplished, he and they know. Yet, I recognize that bright smile and steady gaze of his. There is a certain unparalleled optimism that I've seen shared by many others in the Cochrane fold. I think there is hope if this optimistic group continues to abide by the founding vision and values of the Collaboration – inspired by a jibe from Archie Cochrane – that the future of health care worldwide is only going to be improved by their toil.

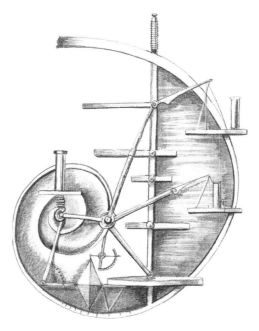

ELEVEN

It's A Start

"Knowledge emerges only through invention and re-invention, through the restless, impatient, continuing, hopeful inquiry human beings pursue in the world, with the world, and with each other."

— Paulo Freire, *Pedagogy of the Oppressed*

THE COCHRANE Collaboration (which has since dropped the word 'Collaboration' from its name) has created a trustworthy brand. In the medical world, people have heard of it and know what it stands for: Trusted Evidence. Informed Decisions. Better Health. At least, that's the latest iteration of its motto. But can we say that Cochrane is making much of a difference?

In seeking an answer to that question, it's worth returning to the maternity ward, where the audacious seed of creating systematic reviews throughout the field of obstetrics took root. From that early and important work in obstetrics, led by Iain Chalmers, Murray Enkin, and a whole host of rebels, an international collaboration has emerged covering most aspects of health care. Even today, the most thoroughly covered area of systematic reviews of healthcare interventions remains pregnancy and childbirth.

Yet, sadly, still too many die. Still too many babies who will never see their first birthday. Still too many babies grow up as orphans of women who die in childbirth.

More than three million newborn babies die every year, and about 287,000 women – about 800 per day, every day – die from preventable causes related to pregnancy and childbirth. The vast majority of those deaths occur in developing countries where poverty, lack of access to health care, and infectious diseases such as HIV and malaria take their toll. Some might say that this is one of the profoundest demonstrations of our collective inhumanity: our inability to halt deaths that arise from humanity's deep urge to bring life into this world.

Yet, others might see reasons for optimism. In 2010, maternal mortality worldwide was almost half what it had been in 1990. In the space of 20 years, we made great strides in improving the lives of people through greater knowledge about how to prevent suffering while bringing new people into the world more humanely. For far too many couples, the day that should be among their happiest – the birth of their child – brings tragedy. But there are many devoting their energies and their passions to change that.

Shaking the System; Creating the Product

Lelia Duley felt that she was about to witness something significant. Yet, in a crowd populated by some of the world's powerhouses in obstetrics and gynecology – as well as other fields of medicine – she wondered why she was there.[134]

"I was just a minnow," she said. She was a junior researcher at the meeting that established the Cochrane Collaboration in Oxford in October, 1993. She felt as if it was "history in the making," and there was a definite buzz in the air.

Another junior researcher at that meeting was a young Croatian obstetrician in training named Zarko Alfirevic. He was studying in Liverpool and was familiar with the relatively new world of systematic reviews in obstetrics and the research contained within the *Oxford Database of Perinatal Trials*. He, too, felt that there was something special about the group of people at that first meeting.[135]

What hooked Alfirevic was the iconoclastic nature of it; the feeling that something completely different was about to happen. Brought up and trained in Croatia, he describes where he came from as a "very rigid, structured system where doctors are never wrong, and where 'Why?' was not really a word that we used." He added, "And then, seeing this group of people who are completely anti-establishment, who think completely differently – that was a shock to my system."

Now a professor at the University of Liverpool, England, Alfirevic is a big fish. He's the co-ordinating editor of the Cochrane Pregnancy and Childbirth Review Group and of a Collaboration that he said has "gone mainstream." In his Croatian accent tinged with British inflections (a legacy of more than two decades in the UK), he speaks of the past with some nostalgia. "I am the very establishment that people are fighting against. I really like and still see myself as a part of this group which was designed to shake the system; not *be* the system."

He blushes a bit when he remembers himself as a brash young researcher, standing up at that meeting and announcing to the assembled group of experts, "Well, it's all very well talking, but I think we just need to go home and just do these reviews, because it's actually what we need. It's the product." He acknowledges how much the Collaboration, its bureaucracy and its institutional needs, have ballooned, but he says he's still attached to this one basic concept that brings everyone together: "It's about the product."

And the products are the reviews: the careful, painstaking hunts through the literature, finding and assessing the quality of research, and pointing out where the gaps are. It's the result when consumers, librarians, researchers, clinicians and statisticians all over the world create something that epitomizes independent, high-quality evidence that people can rely on when they make healthcare decisions.

New Standards for Vision and Ambition

Lelia Duley, the self-professed minnow, had a strong desire to be one of the people who made these products.

When Duley met Iain Chalmers, she was a registrar in obstetrics at the John Radcliffe Hospital in Oxford, England. She went to see him at the National Perinatal Epidemiology Unit and told him that she wanted to become a perinatal epidemiologist (someone who studies how often and why different outcomes happen for mothers and infants around childbirth).

The reception she got might not have been particularly warm. Iain Chalmers remembers meeting her: "We said that she must be mad to take on such an insecure existence and sent her away to ponder what we had said. But she kept on coming back." She eventually got a training fellowship and joined the team.

"Iain asked me to do the first review of anticonvulsants," said Duley, referring to a class of drugs used to help prevent seizures in pregnant women. Eclampsia and its precursor, pre-eclampsia, are characterized by high blood pressure and protein in the urine, and can lead to seizures or convulsions, sometimes coma, and even death.

Of the 300,000-or-so women who die every year around the world from complications of pregnancy and childbirth, about 15 per cent of those deaths are linked to eclampsia. The tragedy, of course, is that many of those deaths are easily preventable.

At the time, in the early 1990s, Duley said, there were few trials and only a handful of agents that showed any promise. Among those were diazepam (Valium), a popular anti-anxiety drug; phenytoin (an anti-epileptic drug); and lytic cocktail (a mixture of sedative and analgesic drugs). The big question was which of those treatments worked best.

Duley went on to design and lead a large trial, the results of which were published in *The Lancet* in 1995. Her team compared diazepam and phenytoin to magnesium sulfate in women with eclampsia.[136] Magnesium sulfate (also known as Epsom salts) is used in medicine in a variety of ways: to treat aches and pains, as a laxative, as an anti-arrhythmia drug, to help treat asthma, and to prevent cerebral palsy following preterm birth. It's an extremely versatile substance that can go a long way in preventing suffering and death. Plus, it's ridiculously cheap.

Duley's collaborative eclampsia trial, coordinated from Oxford, recruited 1,687 women with eclampsia from Africa, India and South America. The trial found that the women treated with magnesium sulfate had a "52% lower risk of recurrent convulsions" when compared to diazepam, a 67% lower risk when compared to phenytoin, and died less frequently. The mothers treated with magnesium sulfate were less likely to develop pneumonia or to be admitted to intensive care facilities than those given phenytoin. She concluded that these findings represented "compelling evidence in favour of magnesium sulfate, rather than diazepam or phenytoin, for the treatment of eclampsia."[137]

Richard Lilford, a notable British epidemiologist and expert on the development of clinical trials, wrote, "Within a year of the publication of Lelia Duley's study, magnesium sulfate use improved from zero to 80 per cent of women in the UK. That was without any guidelines."[138] Lilford called Duley's trial "*the* trial of the 1990s."

In a commentary in the *BMJ*,[139] Jim Neilson went a bit further, describing Duley's trial as "the most important obstetric trial in the 20th century." He also noted that, until then, "the pharmacological treatment of eclampsia [had] been determined largely by geography, habit, and prejudice." He pointed out that magnesium sulfate was the drug of choice in the USA, while British doctors favored diazepam and phenytoin – not because the Americans were any smarter, but because, as he noted, "none of these choices was influenced by strong scientific evidence."

Now there was evidence. Neilson wrote that Duley's trial "set new standards for vision and ambition in clinical trials in perinatal medicine." But there was more work to do.

The Magpie Trial

When I asked Jim Neilson to explain this further he recalled that, in the mid-1990s, even after Duley's trial produced such definitive results, "there was still uncertainty around the benefits of using magnesium sulfate for pre-eclampsia."[140] One might reason that if magnesium sulfate was useful for eclampsia, it might also be useful for pre-eclampsia. He said, "It was being used in North America and parts of South America, but in huge parts of the world (including the UK and Africa), it wasn't being used at all."

So, another much larger trial was launched. It was known as the Magpie Trial[141] and recruited more than 10,000 pregnant women from 33 countries – mostly in Africa, Latin America, and Europe – between July, 1998 and November, 2001. The eligibility criteria: The women had to have pre-eclampsia and "there needed to be uncertainty about whether [or not] to use magnesium sulfate." Most women were recruited while on the labor ward of a hospital. Lelia Duley was the clinical coordinator of the trial.

Her colleague, Jim Neilson, not one for exaggeration, said that Magpie was, "very much a history-making, a really important trial." And again the magnesium sulfate won out. "The risk of eclampsia – seizures and high blood pressure – was reduced by half." He said that when they did a national audit in the UK later, the incidence of pre-eclampsia (because more women were being offered magnesium sulfate) also dropped by half.

Neilson said that Duley went on to be responsible for most of the systematic reviews in pre-eclampsia – dominated by the Magpie trial – which showed clear evidence of benefit. He said that these reviews, "did much to boost the Cochrane brand within the obstetric community."

Systematic Reviews, and Beliefs and Prejudices

Many in the Collaboration have pointed to Duley's work as the quintessential Cochrane output: a clear example of an important question being answered definitively by a systematic review of randomized trials. There is no doubt that the reduction in deaths from eclampsia worldwide can be attributed, at least in part, to the work of Duley and her colleagues.

Yet I wondered what else in the pregnancy and childbirth section of the *Cochrane Library* was making a significant difference in the lives of people in the developing world. I put this question to Jim Neilson.

He didn't hesitate. "One of the most downloaded reviews in the *Cochrane Library* showed that if a pregnant woman has someone with them in labor, there are tangible clinical benefits as well as improved satisfaction all around." He went on to say that women fare better, have fewer cesarean sections, and generally report feeling better if they have some support while in labor. He added, "That support could be [from] anybody. Sometimes it's with a doula; sometimes with midwives providing continuous care."

This seemed blindingly obvious to me, but Neilson said that in large parts of the world women have no companionship during labor, even though "we take it for granted in Europe and North America. It's an intervention that's not a drug and not high tech, but it's terribly important."

He saw it firsthand in Zimbabwe. The hospitals were "unbelievably busy," with people all over the place, but the women admitted to deliver babies were told that they couldn't have their partners or family members with them. He saw it again in the mid-1980s in Malawi, where women going into labor weren't allowed to have companions on the labor ward. He's been back more recently (2012), and noted, "They are definitely trying to change that."

Obviously, local practices, available resources, and other factors form what each culture deems appropriate in giving birth. Even in richer countries, Neilson says, the type of labor support given to women can make a big difference, an outcome supported by Cochrane systematic reviews.

He referred me to Ellen Hodnett, a professor of nursing in Toronto who has worked as an editor in the Pregnancy and Childbirth Group for many years.[142] One of Hodnett's main research areas is "continuous support during childbirth."[143] I asked her, "Isn't it obvious that women who have someone supporting them in labor do better? It would seem that a trial is unethical."

"Not at all," she replied. "Really, this is what is fundamental to what Iain Chalmers would have said about many, many Cochrane reviews. We often examine things that seem to be self-evident. Sometimes they are not, and sometimes they are, but like in the labor-support review, there are usually some qualifications around the results."

She continued, "The overall conclusions of that review are

quite clearly favorable – in terms of increased spontaneous vaginal birth, increased satisfaction, decreased interventions, and so on." Essentially, if you have someone there to help you through labor, you're more likely to have a less technologized, more satisfactory birth.

Her review went on to inform guidelines put out by groups across North America and the UK, such as the Society of Obstetricians and Gynaecologists of Canada, who say that labor support is a pretty good idea. In some countries, delivery support is appalling, and the conditions for giving birth even more so.

Hodnett said, "It's not surprising that under really terrible conditions for women, in developing countries, providing a caring and supportive [companion] is going to make a dramatic difference." Perhaps a testimony to the growing importance of Cochrane reviews, she said that this review helped to support changes in legislation in Brazil and Uruguay, giving women a legal right to support during labor.[144] But all is not perfectly rosy.

Evidence doesn't suddenly transform into practice changes. How it is brought into practice will be as unique as its jurisdiction's particular context. Hodnett said that, when her review came out and guidelines were being changed, "I got a lot of pushback from North American hospitals, who said, 'We can't afford to have nurses providing continuous labor support.'" In other words, the way hospitals were organizing labor and delivery units, staffed by nurses based on "average" workloads, wasn't going to work.

Hodnett explains: "Women don't come in [based upon] averages. The workload is all over the map, [the] nurses were either sitting around with nothing to do, or, they were crazy busy doing everything." So she did what any researcher would do in that situation: she submitted a grant proposal to study things further.

"We got NIH funding to do a trial of 7,000 women in labor

in which our question was this: Is labor support by nurses effective within the typical delivery unit in North American hospitals?"

To do this trial, they had to train nurses in labor support and train the hospitals so that they would staff the delivery support by nurses in hospitals: it didn't make a damned bit of difference. Everything was absolutely the same."[145]

She continued: "It became clear to us why. A great majority of those women had been given oxytocin, continuous fetal monitoring, [intravenous] drugs, and so on. They were confined to bed and strapped to machines." She sighs and adds, "And we expected to see a difference?"

The birth environment is so essential, she says. One factor is that, in many countries, birth is increasingly a high-tech experience, with high intervention rates and high cesarean section rates that, in Hodnett's words, show "no demonstrable benefit for the babies and added risk to the mothers." As a consequence of that study, she had to incorporate the new information into a new Cochrane review: "I had to redo the whole review from the get-go."

I asked her a stark question: So is Cochrane winning the war in terms of more humane and rational approaches to in-hospital childbirth? She pondered for a while. A long while. Then she said, "It wasn't that long ago [that] when you said the words 'Cochrane Review,' most clinicians would look at you blankly. Now it's a given. The awareness is much higher."

But that awareness doesn't always translate into change. When Cochrane reviews support firmly held beliefs, they get adopted. When they don't, they often get criticized instead. She said, "If you take the easier thing – like when I was a labor and delivery nurse in the 1970s, they did routine shaves, preps and enemas. Those things disappeared pretty quickly. You could argue that nobody needed a Cochrane review to say, 'This is stupid.'"

Yet other things continue, some of which also seem pretty

stupid. "We still have continuous electronic fetal monitoring, and it's pretty stupid," she says. But "evidence-based care is more complex than just knowing the evidence and adopting it."

Zarko Alfirevic agrees with this sentiment. He points to one of his reviews of the umbilical arterial Doppler,[146] an ultrasound test used in high-risk pregnancies. "It basically targets a vessel that connects the placenta with the baby. By looking at the pattern of blood flow from [the] placenta into the baby, we can predict – or we think that we can predict – whether this is a pregnancy that needs to be delivered sooner or if it's safe to continue.

"So, we did it as a Cochrane review, and then published it in the *American Journal of Obstetrics and Gynecology*," he said. That review has had pretty good staying power. "It's one of the [most] highly quoted papers or pieces of work that I have been involved with. But interestingly, it was only so because it had a positive message, that the test was beneficial. We have since published or [done] many other reviews that had an equally powerful, if not more powerful, message that the things, or the tests, don't work." Those negative reviews, he said, have had "nowhere near the impact."

Epilogue

IT'S A fitting conclusion to this book. Alfirevic summarizes the predicament saying, "To this day, I find this absolutely fascinating how we as a medical profession are absolutely in love with the treatments, with anything that kind of works or is statistically significant, and just can't cope when something that is close to our heart doesn't work, or somebody dares to say that there is not enough evidence [for it]."

Is it just a simple case of attacking or praising the messenger? That's part of it. Many times, when the evidence that comes out of a systematic review is controversial, one's tendency to attack or to praise the Cochrane Collaboration will depend on your existing beliefs and prejudices.

How does Alfirevic feel about this state of affairs? "That's life... and on one level I feel actually quite proud about it because... 20 years ago very few people... 'got it.' Now, it is quite rewarding that not every lecture or discussion about evidence has to start with a 15-minute introduction of what is Cochrane, what is a forest plot, and so on." He adds, "People now kind of get it. Most people do."

There is still an unbearable amount of death and suffering related to childbirth in this world. Too many women and their babies suffer and die needlessly, often victims of poverty and neglect. To many diseases, like those suffered by Chris Silagy or Alessandro Liberati are crying out for proper research to help doctors and patients make decisions, but that research is almost non-existent. At the same time, the body of high-quality systematic reviews produced by the Cochrane Collaboration continues to grow. Thousands of people around the world are doing what they can, contributing to the conversation about what works and what doesn't.

Around the world there are millions of women going into labor whose care has been influenced by the likes of Duley, Neilson, Hodnett and Alfirevic.

Is it enough? No, it isn't. Is it a start? Yes, it's a solid start.

Acknowledgements

FOR THE thousands of people who work under the banner of Cochrane, you deserve the most acknowledgement, for without your efforts, the Cochrane Library would simply not exist, and modern health care would be much poorer.

The biggest thanks go to the nearly 160 people both inside and outside the Cochrane Collaboration (many of whom are listed below) who agreed to spend time answering my questions in person, or by phone, skype or email. I thank you very much and I want you to know that even if you don't find your story in this book, everything I heard, read, saw or otherwise absorbed about this organization is reflected in the manuscript.

Several key people were notably helpful and supportive, especially (and in no particular order) Iain Chalmers, Murray Enkin, Jini Hetherington, Nancy Owens, Jeremy Grimshaw, David Tovey, Don Husereau, Marc Christensen, Andrew Macleod, Kay Dickersin, Peter Gøtzsche, and Maryanne Napoli. To my wife Lynda and children Morgan and Chase, your tolerance for my disappearances as I wrote this book has been incredible. I have had a lot of editorial help along the way, and particular thanks go to Glenn Harrington and Catherine Plear. Any mistakes are mine and mine alone. Since I know many Cochranites are fastidious nitpickers, and will find things in this book that will drive you crazy, please let me know. If you discover anything that needs to be corrected for future editions, don't hesitate to contact me: cassels@uvic.ca

Individuals interviewed for this book

Adams, Clive
Ahn, Hyeong Sik
Aja, Godwin
Alfirevic, Zarko
Allen, Claire
Altman, Doug
Antes, Gerd
Aronson, Jeffrey
Atallah, Alvaro
Bastian, Hilda
Becker, Lorne
Bell, Warren
Bell-Syer, Sally
Bero, Lisa
Binder, Lucie
Bishop Velarde, Alina
Bonfill, Xavier
Boruch, Bob
Burnand, Bernard
Burton, Martin
Cates, Christopher
Cepeda-Hodgson, Martha
Chalmers, Francie
Chalmers, Iain
Chalmers, Jan
Chandler, Jackie
Clarke, Mike
Clarkson, Jan
Collins, Rory
Craig, Jonathan
Crowley, Patricia
Cuervo, Luis Gabriel
Cumpston, Miranda
Davoli, Marina
Deeks, Jon

Dellavalle, Robert
Dickersin, Kay
Dooley, Gordon
Dormuth, Colin
Duley, Lelia
Durieux, Pierre
Ebrahim, Shah
Enkin, Eleanor
Enkin, Murray
Farquhar, Cindy
Filippini, Graziella
Foxlee, Ruth
Fuller, Colleen
Garner, Paul
Glaziou, Paul
Gøtzsche, Peter
Gray, Muir
Gregory, Daisy
Grimshaw, Jeremy
Guyatt, Gordon
Gyte, Gill
Haines, Andy
Henderson, Sonja
Henry, David
Herxheimer, Andrew
Hetherington, Jini
Higgins, Julian
Hill, Sophie
Hodnett, Ellen
Hopewell, Sally
Hudson, Rick
Husereau, Don
Jadad, Alejandro
Jauca, Ciprian
Jefferson, Tom

Kayabu, Bonnix
Kjeldstrøm, Monica
Kleijnen, Jos
Koretz, Ron
Langhorne, Peter
Lefebvre, Carol
Li, Youping
Liberati, Alessandro
Lumbiganon, Pisake
Macleod, Andrew
Macleod, Stuart
Maclure, Malcolm
Mavergames, Christopher
McDonald, Steve
McDowell, Nicola
McIlwain, Catherine
Middleton, Philippa
Moynihan, Ray
Nabhan, Ashraf
Neilson, Jim
Napoli, Maryann
Nasser, Mona
Noyes, Jane
Okebe, Joseph
Owens, Nancy
Oxman, Andy
Patriarche, Kerry
Pentesco-Gilbert, Deborah
Pérez Koehlmoos, Tracey
Ravaud, Philippe
Reiger, Kareen
Richter, Bernd
Ried, Juliane
Riis, Jacob
Rouse, Caroline

Rowe, Brian
Sackett, Barbara
Sackett, Dave
Salanti, Georgia
Sambunjak, Dario
Schaafsma, Mary-Ellen
Scholten, Robert
Simi, Silvana
Skoetz, Nicole
Soares-Weiser, Karla
Soll, Roger
Stanley, Dana
Starr, Mark
Stead, Lindsay
Tarbett, Lori
Tharyan, Prathap
Thomas, Jessica
Tovey, David
Tristan, Mario
Tugwell, Peter
Urrutia, Gerard
Vasumathi, Sriganesh
Verbeek, Jos
Volmink, Jimmy
Wale, Janet
Walsh, Marilyn
Waters, Elizabeth
Weatherall, David
Whamond, Liz
Worthington, Helen
Wright, Jim
Zhang, Mingming

ENDNOTES

1 Cochrane AL: *Effectiveness and Efficiency: Random Reflections on Health Services.* London: Nuffield Provincial Hospitals Trust, 1972.

2 Pratt EJ: *Complete Poems*, ed. Sandra Djwa and RG Moyles. Toronto: University of Toronto Press, 1989.

3 I interviewed Nancy Owens on October 19, 2011 in Madrid, Spain. Over the course of my writing this book, Nancy and I have had many more conversations and have frequently communicated by email.

4 In the December 2012 edition of *The Cochrane Library*, there are 99 hits for the word "colorectal" that include all kinds of therapies, surgical techniques, and drugs related to the treatment of colorectal cancer.

5 I interviewed Kay Dickersin on October 19, 2011 in Madrid, Spain. I have kemt in touch with her by email and frequently see her at international conventions.

6 Rettig R et al: *False Hope: Bone Marrow Transplantation for Breast Cancer.* Oxford: Oxford University Press, 2007.

7 Dickersin K, Straus SE, and Bero LA: "Medical Milestones," *BMJ* 334 (Jan. 2007), www.bmj.com/highwire/filestream/438857/field_highwire_adjunct_files/0.

8 Smith SE: "Pinkification: How Breast Cancer Awareness Got Commodified for Profit," *Guardian Comment Network* (Oct. 3, 2012), www.guardian.co.uk/commentisfree/2012/oct/03/pinkification-breast-cancer-awareness-commodified.

9 Advertisement in *Mother Jones*, Jan. 1990.

10 www.breastcancer.org/symptoms/understand_bc/statistics.

11 I interviewed Peter Gøtzsche on October 21, 2011 in Madrid, Spain. Over the course of my writing this book, Peter and I have had many more conversations.

12 Gøtzsche P: "Time to Stop Mammography?" *CMAJ* 183, no. 17 (Nov. 22, 2011), www.cmaj.ca/content/183/17/1957.full.

13 Author's interview with Iain Chalmers, Oxford, UK. April 13, 2012.

14 Cassels A: *Seeking Sickness: Medical Screening and the Misguided Hunt for Disease.* Vancouver: Greystone, 2012. p. 43. USPSTF, Prostate Cancer Screening Recommendation Summary, May 2012. www.uspreventiveservicestaskforce.org/Page/Topic/recommendation-summary/prostate-cancer-screening

15 Prochazka AV and Caverly T: "General Health Checks in Adults for Reducing Morbitity and Mortality from Disease: Summary Review of Primary Findings and Conclusions," *JAMA Internal Medicine* Jan 14, 2013, citations 7 and 8.

16 Chalmers I, in the 1999 edition foreword to Cochrane AL: *Effectiveness and Efficiency: Random Reflections on Health Services.* London: Nuffield Provincial Hospitals Trust, 1972. Reprinted in 1989 in association with the *BMJ.* Reprinted in 1999 for Nuffield Trust by the Royal Society of Medicine Press, London (ISBN 1-85315-394-X). p xiii.

17 I interviewed Iain Chalmers on April 13, 2012 at his office in Oxford. Over the course of my writing this book, Iain and I have had many more conversations by telephone and by skype.

18 Cochrane AL: *Effectiveness and Efficiency: Random Reflections on Health Services.* London: Nuffield Provincial Hospitals Trust, 1972.

19 ibid, p. 4.

20 ibid, p. xiii.

21 Cochrane AL: Extracts from "Sickness in Salonica: My First, Worst, and Most Successful Clinical Trial." *BM J* 289: 1726–27 (1984).

22 Cochrane AL: *Effectiveness and Efficiency: Random Reflections on Health Services.* London: Nuffield Provincial Hospitals Trust, 1972, p 6.

23 Interview with Iain Chalmers in Oxford. Oct 13, 2012.

24 Cochrane AL: "1931–1971: A Critical Review with Particular Reference to the Medical Profession" *Medicines for the Year 2000.* London: Office of Health Economics, (1979) pp 1–11.

25 Chalmers I: "Archie Cochrane (1909-1988)" (an essay in the James Lind Library), 2006. www.jameslindlibrary.org/illustrating/articles/archie-cochrane-1909-1988

26 I interviewed Jan Chalmers in Oxford, April, 2012.

27 I interviewed Murray and Eleanor Enkin in Victoria, Canada, May 3, 2012 and have since visited them at their home on many occasions.

28   Chard T and Richards M: "Benefits and Hazards of the New Obstetrics"
     Clinics in Developmental Medicine Series, Vol. 64. London: Heinemann,
     1977.

29   Chalmers I, Enkin M, and Keirse M: *Effective Care in Pregnancy and
     Childbirth, volumes I and II.* London: Oxford University Press, 1989.

30   Chalmers I (ed.): *Oxford Database of Perinatal Trials* (software). Oxford:
     Oxford University Press, 1986.

31   Chalmers I et al. *A Guide to Effective Care in Pregnancy and Childbirth.*
     Oxford: Oxford University Press, 1989.

32   Sinclair JC et al: *Effective Care of the Newborn Infant.* Oxford: Oxford
     University Press, 1992.

33   Fox DM: "Systematic Reviews and Health Policy: The
     Influence of A Project on Perinatal Care Since 1988." *JLL
     Bulletin: Commentaries On The History Of Treatment Evaluation*
     (2011). Co-published in *The Milbank Quarterly* 2011, 89:
     425–449. www.jameslindlibrary.org/illustrating/articles/
     systematic-reviews-and-health-policy-the-influence-of-a-projec

34   Fox, ibid.

35   I formally interviewed Jini Hetherington in Madrid, Oct 19, 2011. In
     the course of writing this book, I have spoken with her, exchanged emails
     and had skype calls on many occasions. She is the Jini mentioned in the
     dedication.

36   Cochrane AL (foreword): Chalmers I, Enkin M and Keirse M eds:
     "Effective Care in Pregnancy and Childbirth," *MJNC.* Oxford: Oxford
     University Press, 1989.

37   No author listed: "Evidence-based Medicine, in Its Place" *Lancet* 346
     (8978): 785 (Sep 23, 1995). This is the same editorial that David Sackett
     refers to when talking about the language of discrimination applied to
     evidence-based medicine.

38   I interviewed Muir Gray in Oxford on April 13, 2012.

39   Attributed to Muir Gray.

40   Chalmers I, Dickersin K, and Chalmers TC: "Getting to Grips with
     Archie Cochrane's Agenda" *BMJ* 1992 305(6857): 786–788.

41   Chalmers I in *Archie Cochrane: Back To The Front* by F. Xavier Bosch, p
     250, Francis Xavier Bosch, 2003.

42   I interviewed Monica Kjeldstrøm by skype on January 7, 2013 from her
     offices in Copenhagen. She died on October 19, 2014.

43 This is referred to in Cochrane literature as the Danish National Theatre.

44 I interviewed Mark Starr by skype from his home in Oxford on April 30, 2012.

45 I travelled with my good friend Don Husereau to Irish Lake, north of Toronto to interview David Sackett at his home on October 31, 2012. Since it was Halloween, and knowing that Sackett liked Kurt Vonnegut, Don dressed as Billy Pilgrim, a World War II soldier, and the main character in Kurt Vonnegut's novel *Slaughterhouse Five*. Sackett died on May 13, 2015 in his 81st year.

46 No author listed: "Evidence-based Medicine, in Its Place" *Lancet*. 346 (8978): 785 (Sep 23, 1995).

47 I interviewed Dr. Francie Chalmers, who lives and works just outside of Seattle, by telephone on October 26, 2012.

48 Interview with Malcolm Maclure, Dr. Tom Chalmers: "The Trials of a Randomizer" *CMAJ* 155 (6) 16 Sep, 1996, 1917-1995.

49 ibid.

50 I interviewed Sir Rory Collins in Oxford on April 13, 2012.

51 "Evidence Updates" BMJ Group and McMaster University's Health Information Research Unit: www.plus.mcmaster.ca/evidenceupdates/ This web resource is to "provide you with access to current best evidence from research, tailored to your own health care interests, to support evidence-based clinical decisions. It takes all citations (from over 120 premier clinical journals) pre-rated for quality by research staff, then they are "rated for clinical relevance and interest by at least 3 members of a worldwide panel of practicing physicians."

52 I interviewed Hilda Bastian on Oct 20, 211 in Madrid. I have conversed with her many times since, and received a huge amount of supporting material, notes, and explanations via e-mail.

53 Cartoon in *Cochrane News* 6, Feb, 1996. www.cochrane.org/sites/default/files/uploads/cochrane_news/CochraneNews-issue6.PDF

54 I interviewed Jini Hetherington in Madrid, Oct 19, 2011.

55 I interviewed Kay Dickersin in Madrid on Oct 19, 2011. I have communicated with her many times since by phone and by e-mail.

56 Though I never got a chance to interview Chris Silagy, it was easy to get a measure of his influence by reading his writings and interviewing a number of the Australians who worked alongside him in the mid-1990s.

57 Much of what I constructed about Chris Silagy comes from his writings and from interviews with Sally Green, Steve McDonald, and Caroline Crowther.

58 Silagy C: "The Post-Cochrane Agenda: Consumers and Evidence" in: Cochrane, AL: *Effectiveness and Efficiency: Random Reflections on Health Services*. London: Royal Society of Medicine Press/Nuffield Trust, 1999, p xxvii.

59 On December 14, 2001, Iain Chalmers wrote a poignant letter to the *BMJ* entitled "The Cochrane Collaboration's debt to Chris Silagy" found at: www.bmj.com/rapid-response/2011/10/28/cochrane-collaborations-debt-chris-silagy and Chalmers' words come from that letter.

60 Dave Sackett is well-remembered by his friends and colleagues. The last series of interviews he gave can be accessed here: www.fhs.mcmaster.ca/ceb/docs/David_L_Sackett_Interview_in_2014_2015.pdf

61 Healy M: "More than 1 in 10 babies worldwide born prematurely" *USA Today*, May 3,2012. http://usatoday30.usatoday.com/news/health/story/2012-05-02/CDC-preterm-premature-births/54692356/1

62 World Health Organization; March of Dimes; The Partnership for Maternal, Newborn & Child Health; Save the Children: *Born Too Soon: the Global Action Report on Preterm Birth*, New York, May 2,2012.

    www.who.int/pmnch/media/news/2012/preterm_birth_report/en/

63 Ki-moon B: Foreword. *Born Too Soon: the global action report on preterm birth*. 2012.

    www.who.int/maternal_child_adolescent/documents/born_too_soon/en/index.html

64 Reynolds LA and Tansey EM: "Prenatal Corticosteroids for Reducing Morbidity and Mortality After Preterm Birth," the transcript of a witness seminar held by the Wellcome Trust Centre for the History of Medicine at UCL, London on June 15, 2004. Letter from Mont Liggins dated April 6, 2004.

65 Obituary of Graham Mont Liggins, *The Guardian*, Sep 6, 2010. www.history.qmul.ac.uk/research/modbiomed/Publications/wit_vols/44848.pdfhttp://www.guardian.co.uk/society/2010/sep/06/sir-graham-mont-liggins-obituary

66 ibid.

67 Reynolds and Tansey, p. 87

68 Watts G: obituary for GC Liggins, *The Lancet* 2010, 376
(9747): 1140 www.thelancet.com/journals/lancet/article/
PIIS0140-6736(10)61528-0/fulltext

69 Liggins GC and Howie RN: "A Controlled Trial of Antepartum
Glucocorticoid Treatment for Prevention of The Respiratory Distress
Syndrome in Premature Infants," *Pediatrics,* 1972; 50(4): 515–25.

70 I interviewed Patricia Crowley by skype on Dec 3, 2012

71 Chalmers I, Enkin M, and Keirse MJ: *Effective Care in Pregnancy and
Childbirth,* Oxford: Oxford University Press, 1989.

72 I interviewed Roger Soll in Paris on April 17, 2012 and had subsequent
telephone conversations with him to record the details as expressed in
this chapter.

73 Sinclair JC, Bracken MB, Silverman W, eds: *Effective Care of the Newborn
Infant.* Oxford: Oxford University Press, 1992.

74 Crowley P, Chalmers I, and Keirse MJ: "The Effects of Corticosteroid
Administration before Preterm Delivery: An Overview of the Evidence
from Controlled Trials," *BJOG,* 1990; 97(1):11–25. [PubMed] Crowley
P. Prophylactic corticosteroids for preterm birth. *Cochrane Database Syst
Rev* 2002; (4): CD000065.

75 Spock B: *Common Sense Book of Baby and Child Care.* Duell, New York:
Sloan and Pearce, 1946.

76 Guntheroth, WG and Spiers, PS: "Infant Sleeping Position and Sudden
Infant Death Syndrome: A Systematic Review," Intl J Epidemiol
2005;34:1165-66.

77 I interviewed Maryann Napoli on October 21, 2011 in Madrid. I have
known her for many years and have had numerous discussions with her,
mostly at past Cochrane colloquia.

78 The term "consumer" essentially means the general public, the consumers
of medical care. Consumer involvement has always been a contentious
and highly debated issue in Cochrane. A survey of consumers conducted
in 2015 reported the following: "Overall, the review concludes that
Cochrane pioneered the involvement of consumers in research and pres-
ently there are over 1,330 Archie registered Consumers, with an active
core of between 300 and 500 regularly involved in the production of
health evidence. This is something to celebrate; however practice across
Cochrane varies and, with some notable exceptions, it has not kept pace
with the world outside Cochrane. Review Groups and Consumers are
looking for support to develop practice in involvement." The survey is
reported at: http://consumers.cochrane.org/news/feature-story

79 I interviewed David Tovey on October 23, 2011 in Madrid. I have since had numerous contacts with him by skype and by e-mail.

80 I interviewed Silvana Simi on October 22, 2011 in Madrid. I have also known her for many years and met her many times at Cochrane colloquia.

81 Higgins JPT and Green S, eds: *Cochrane Handbook for Systematic Reviews of Interventions.* Version 5.1.0 [updated March 2011]. The Cochrane Collaboration; 2011. Available from www.cochrane-handbook.org

82 I interviewed Godwin Aja on April 17, 2012 in Paris.

83 UN Millenium Project: *Global Burden of Malaria.* www.unmillennium-project.org/documents/GlobalBurdenofMalaria.pdf

84 I interviewed Mingming Zhang in Madrid on October 22, 2011.

85 I interviewed Alina Bishop Velarde in Madrid on October 21, 2011.

86 Olsen O and Clausen JA: *Planned Hospital Birth Versus Planned Home Birth.* Cochrane Pregnancy and Childbirth Group. Published online: Sep, 2012. http://onlinelibrary.wiley.com/doi/10.1002/14651858.CD000352.pub2/abstract

87 UN General Assembly factsheet on GOAL 5: Improve Maternal Health www.un.org/millenniumgoals/pdf/MDG_FS_5_EN_new.pdf

88 Chalmers I: "Unbiased, Relevant, and Reliable Assessment in Health Care," *BMJ* 1998; 317: 1167–1168.

89 Kaiser L, Wat C, Mills T, Mahoney P, Ward P, and Hayden F: "Impact of Oseltamivir Treatment on Influenza-Related Lower Respiratory Tract Complications and Hospitalizations," *Arch Intern Med J* (2003) 163, 1667-1672.

90 Jefferson T: Open Knowledge Foundation Blog (2012), http://blog.okfn.org/2012/11/19/the-tamiflu-story-why-we-need-access-to-all-data-from-clinical-trials/.

91 Kmietowicz Z: "Roche Should Be Sued to Release Data on Oseltamivir, Says Cochrane Leader," *BMJ* 345 (2012), published Nov 12, 2012, e7658.

92 Payne D: "Tamiflu: The Battle for Secret Drug Data," BMJ (2012) 345: e7303, Oct 29, 2012 www.bmj.com/content/345/bmj.e7303#ref-4

93 BMJ 2014;348:g2695 www.bmj.com/content/bmj/348/bmj.g2695.full.pdf

94 Chalmers I: "Underreporting Research Is Scientific Misconduct," *JAMA* 263(10), 1405-1408. doi:10.1001/jama.1990.03440100121018. Mar 9, 1990 http://jama.jamanetwork.com/article.aspx?articleid=380971.

95 Chalmers I: *Open Letter to Roche about Oseltamivir Trial Data: Letter to Sir John Bell*, Nov 9, 2012. www.bmj.com/content/345/bmj.e7305/ rr/613849

96 Jefferson T et al.: Letter from Tom Jefferson and Colleagues to Alexis Bicknell, Senior PR Executive, Roche Products Limited, Nov 8, 2012, accessed on the *BMJ* website at www.bmj.com//tamiflu/roche/rr/613652.

97 Angell M: "Is Academic Medicine for Sale?" *NEJM* 2000; 343:508-510 Aug 17, 2000.

98 I formally interviewed Peter Gotzsche on Oct 21, 2011 in Madrid, but have also spoken to him by telephone, by skype, and at conferences numerous times since. When this chapter was originally written, he had just published his book on mammography called *Mammography Screening: Truth, Lies and Controversy*. In 2013, he published *Deadly Medicines and Organised Crime: How Big Pharma has Corrupted Healthcare*. His latest book, on psychiatry, was published in 2015.

99 Jørgensen AW, Hilden J, and Gøtzsche PC: *Cochrane Reviews Compared with Industry Supported Meta-analyses and Other Meta-analyses of The Same Drugs: Systematic Review* doi:10.1136/bmj.38973.444699.0B Oct 6, 2006. www.bmj.com/content/333/7572/782?tab=responses

100 I initially interviewed Lisa Bero at the Loon Lake Research & Education Centre outside of Vancouver on Mar 28, 2012; and later by telephone from her office in San Francisco on Sep 4, 2012. I have known Lisa for many years and we have discussed our research, the Cochrane Collaboration, and many other issues before and since then. She is now one of the Co-chairs of the Cochrane Collaboration and teaches at the University of Sydney, in Sydney Australia.

101 I interviewed Ron Koretz by telephone on Sep 25, 2012. He is an Emeritus Professor of Clinical Medicine at the UCLA School of Medicine.

102 I met Ray Moynihan in 2001 after he had published an important study on the quality of medical journalism. We became collaborators, co-authors on a bestselling book called *Selling Sickness* (2005), and friends. I consider him one of my closest mentors.

103 Moynihan R: "Cochrane at Crossroads over Drug Company Sponsorship," *BMJ* Oct 18, 200 3327(7420): 924–926.

104 I interviewed Jim Neilson on Nov 29, 2012 by skype from the Liverpool Women's Hospital, Liverpool.

105 Roseman M, Turner EH, Lexchin J, Coyne JC, Bero L, and Thombs BD: "Reporting of conflicts of interest from drug trials in Cochrane reviews: cross sectional study," *BMJ* 345 (2012), doi: http://dx.doi.org/10.1136/bmj.e5155 (Published August 21, 2012) e5155: http://www.bmj.com/content/345/bmj.e5155.

106 Bero L: "Why the Cochrane risk of bias tool should include funding source as a standard item" [editorial]. Cochrane Database of Systematic Reviews 2013;(12): 10.1002/14651858.ED000075. Her commentary can be found at: www.cochranelibrary.com/editorial/10.1002/14651858.ED000075

107 I interviewed Mike Clark on Oct 20, 2011 in Madrid.

108 *Cochrane Gem* for the week of Jan 4, 2005, written by "Insider." It can be found here: http://laikaspoetnik.wordpress.com/2010/01/24/cochrane-evidence-aid-for-catastrophes-like-haitis-earthquake-helping-by-doing-what-we-do-best/

109 Tharyan P, Clarke M, and Green S: "How the Cochrane Collaboration Is Responding to The Asian Tsunami." *PLOS Med.* 2005; 2(6): e169.

110 I interviewed Bonnix Kayabu on Oct 19, 2011 in Madrid.

111 I interviewed Prathap Tharyan on Oct 22, 2011 in Madrid.

112 McKnight J: *The Careless Society: Community and Its Counterfeits*. New York: Basic Books, 1995.

113 As reported in Laika's blog at: http://laikaspoetnik.wordpress.com/2010/01/24/cochrane-evidence-aid-for-catastrophes-like-haitis-earthquake-helping-by-doing-what-we-do-best/

114 Tharyan P, Clarke M, and Green S: "How the Cochrane Collaboration Is Responding to The Asian Tsunami." PLOS Med. 2005; 2(6): e169.

115 Committee on the Learning Health Care System in America; Institute of Medicine; Smith M, Saunders R, Stuckhardt L et al, eds: *Best Care at Lower Cost: The Path to Continuously Learning Health Care in America*. Washington: National Academies Press (US), May 10, 2013.

116 Brownlee S: *Overtreated: Why Too Much Medicine Is Making Us Poorer and Sicker*. New York: Bloomsbury USA; 2007.

117 Institute of Medicine website: www.iom.edu/About-IOM.aspx

118 Institute of Medicine: *The Healthcare Imperative: Lowering Costs And Improving Outcomes*, 2010;

Ellis P et al: "Wide Variation in Episode Costs within A Commercially Insured Population Highlights Potential To Improve The Efficiency of Care". *Health Affairs*, 2012; 31(9): 2084–93;

Institute of Medicine: *"Best Care at Lower Cost: the path to continuously learning health care in America"* Sep 6, 2012

119 www.iom.edu/Reports/2012/Best-Care-at-Lower-Cost-The-Path-to-Continuously-Learning-Health-Care-in-America.aspx.

120 I met Andrew Herxheimer about 20 years ago, at a meeting with Health Action International in Amsterdam and have been aware of his work ever since. For this book, I interviewed him in Madrid on Oct 21, 2011.

121 I consider Barbara Mintzes a close personal friend and colleague. We have worked together on numerous studies and projects since 1994. She was formerly a member of the Therapeutics Initiative at UBC, the home of the Cochrane Collaboration's Hypertension review group. She now works in Sydney, Australia.

122 Koretz RL, Pleguezuelo M, Arvaniti V, Barrera Baena P, Ciria R, Gurusamy KS, Davidson BR, and Burroughs AK: "Interferon for Interferon Nonresponding and Relapsing Patients with Chronic Hepatitis C," *Cochrane Database of Systematic Reviews*. 2013; CD003617. DOI: 10.1002/14651858.CD003617.pub2.

123 I interviewed Andy Haines on Oct 21, 2011 in Madrid.

124 I interviewed Bob Dellavalle in Madrid on Oct 20, 2011 in Madrid.

125 I interviewed Bob Boruch by telephone on Jan 29, 2013.

126 Dunn WD: *The Experimenting Society: Essays in Honor of Donald T. Campbell*. Piscataway NJ: Transaction Publishers, 1997. https://books.google.ca/books?id=TDuXdlxjdSsC&pg=PA35&hl=en#v=onepage&q&f=true

127 As per my phone conversation with Bob Boruch on Jan 29, 2013.

128 Petrosino A, Turpin-Petrosino C, and Buehler J: "Scared Straight and Other

Juvenile Awareness Programs for Preventing Juvenile Delinquency," *Campbell Systematic Reviews*. 2004:2. DOI: 10.4073/csr.2004.2

129 Tovey D and Dellavalle R: "Cochrane in the United States of America" [editorial]. *Cochrane Database of Systematic Reviews*, 2010. www.cochranelibrary.com/editorial/10.1002/14651858.ED000010

130 ibid.

131 Goldacre B: Foreword to Evans I, Thornton H, Chalmers I, et al: *Testing Treatments: Better Research for Better Healthcare* 2nd edition. London: Pinter & Martin; 2011. www.ncbi.nlm.nih.gov/books/NBK66212/

132 I interviewed Paul Garner on Oct 21, 2011 in Madrid.

133 I Interviewed Jimmy Volmink on April 18, 2012 in Paris.

134 I interviewed Lelia Duley on July 5, 2012 by telephone from her office in Nottingham.

135 I interviewed Zarko Alfirevic on April 17, 2012 in Paris.

136 The Eclampsia Trial Collaborative Group: "Which Anticonvulsant for Women with Eclampsia? Evidence from The Collaborative Eclampsia Trial." *The Lancet.* 1995; 345(8963):1455–63. DOI: 10.1016/S0140-6736(95)91034-4. www.thelancet.com/journals/lancet/article/PIIS0140-6736(95)91034-4/abstract

137 Duley L: "Magnesium Sulphate in Eclampsia," *The Lancet.* 1998; 352(9121): 67–8.

138 Reynolds LA and Tansey EM: "Prenatal Corticosteroids for Reducing Morbidity And Mortality after Preterm Birth." The transcript of a Witness Seminar held by the Wellcome Trust Centre for the History of Medicine at UCL, London. June 15, 2004; p. 61 (said by Liliford).

http://www.history.qmul.ac.uk/research/modbiomed/Publications/wit_vols/44848.pdf

139 Neilson JP: "Magnesium Sulphate: The Drug Of Choice in Eclampsia." *BMJ,* 1995; 311:702 www.bmj.com/content/311/7007/702.

140 I interviewed Jim Neilson on Nov 29, 2012 by skype from his office in Liverpool.

141 The Magpie Trial Collaborative Group: "Do Women with Pre-Eclampsia, and Their Babies, Benefit from Magnesium Sulphate? The Magpie Trial: A Randomised Placebo-Controlled Trial." *The Lancet.* 2002; 359: 1877–90.

142 I interviewed Ellen Hodnett by skype on Dec 4, 2012 from her office in Toronto.

143 Hodnett ED, Gates S, Hofmeyr GJ, and Sakala C: "Continuous Support for Women During Childbirth," Cochrane Database of Systematic Reviews 2012; Issue 10; Art. No.: CD003766. DOI: 10.1002/14651858.CD003766.pub4. http://onlinelibrary.wiley.com/doi/10.1002/14651858.CD003766.pub4/abstract

144 Pedwell S: "Nursing Researcher Talks About Her Work, Childbirth and Labor,". *U of T News*: www.news.utoronto.ca/ nursing-researcher-talks-about-her-work-childbirth-and-labor

145 Hodnett ED, Lowe NK, Hannah ME, Willan AR, Stevens B, Weston JA, Ohlsson A, Gafni A, Muir HA, Myhr TL, and Stremler R: "Nursing Supportive Care in Labor Trial Group. Effectiveness of Nurses As Providers of Birth Labor Support in North American Hospitals: A Randomized Controlled Trial," *JAMA* 2002; 18;288(11):1373–81.

146 Alfirevic Z and Neilson JP: "Doppler ultrasound for fetal assessment in high risk pregnancies," *Cochrane Database of Systematic Reviews*, 2010; Issue 1; Art. No.: CD000073. DOI: 10.1002/14651858.CD000073. pub2.

ABOUT THE AUTHOR
Alan Cassels, CD, MPA

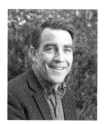

ALAN CASSELS has been immersed in pharmaceutical policy research for the past 20 years, studying how prescription drugs are regulated, marketed, prescribed and used. His books include *Selling Sickness: How the World's Biggest Pharmaceutical Companies are Turning Us All into Patients* (co-written with Ray Moynihan); *The ABCs of Disease Mongering: An Epidemic in 26 Letters*; and *Seeking Sickness: Medical Screening and the Misguided Hunt for Disease.*

In all of his books, Cassels weighs in on the folly of practitioners and profiteers increasingly selling us tests, treatments and theories of disease that threaten to turn more and more of us into patients. He believes that humans need clean information as urgently as they need clean water, and one of the best ways to steer clear of avoidable medical intervention, folly and harm is by using the products of the Cochrane Collaboration, one of the world's best sources of quality medical information.

Cassels is a health policy researcher affiliated with the Faculty of Human and Social Development at the University of Victoria. He is a media commentator on medical policy issues and a frequent contributor to magazines, newspapers and the CBC Radio program *IDEAS*. He lectures and presents keynote speeches around the world.

Contact him at cassels@uvic.ca, twitter: @AKECassels

Made in the USA
Monee, IL
24 March 2024

55677818R00125